High-Yield Obstetrics and Gynecology
2nd edition

High–Yield Obstetrics and Gynecology

2nd edition

Elmar P. Sakala, M.D., M.A., M.P.H.

Professor of Gynecology and Obstetrics

Department of Gynecology and Obstetrics

School of Medicine

Loma Linda University

Loma Linda, California

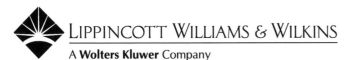

LIPPINCOTT WILLIAMS & WILKINS

A **Wolters Kluwer** Company

Philadelphia · Baltimore · New York · London
Buenos Aires · Hong Kong · Sydney · Tokyo

Acquisitions Editor: Donna Balado
Development Editor: Emilie Linkins
Managing Editor: Elena Coler
Project Editor: Julie Montalbano
Illustrator: Holly R. Fischer

351 West Camden Street
Baltimore, Maryland 21201-2436 USA

530 Walnut Street
Philadelphia, Pennsylvania 19106 USA

First Edition, 2001

Printed in the United States of America

Library of Congress Cataloging-in-Publication Data

Sakala, Elmar P.
  High-yield obstetrics and gynecology / Elmar P. Sakala.—2nd ed.
    p. ; cm.
  Includes index.
  ISBN 13: 978-0-7817-9630-9
  ISBN 10: 0-7817-9630-X
  1. Pregnancy—Examinations, questions, etc. 2. Gynecology—Examinations, questions, etc. 3. Pregnancy—Outlines, syllabi, etc. 4. Gynecology—Outlines, syllabi, etc. I. Title.
  [DNLM: 1. Pregnancy Complications—Examination Questions. 2. Pregnancy Complications—Outlines. 3. Genital Diseases, Female—Examination Questions. 4. Genital Diseases, Female—Outlines. 5. Prenatal Care—Examination Questions. 6. Prenatal Care—Outlines. WQ 18.2 S158h 2005]
  RG524.S24 2005
  618'.07—dc22   2005040925

                                                                              10
                                                              3 4 5 6 7 8 9 10

Dedication

To my wife, Darilee

A wife of noble character who can find?
She is worth far more than rubies.
Her husband has full confidence in her
and lacks nothing of value.
She brings him good, not harm,
all the days of her life.
She speaks with wisdom,
and faithful instruction is on her tongue.
Her children arise and call her blessed:
her husband also, and he praises her.

—from the Proverbs of King Solomon

Preface

It is truly a daunting challenge to cope successfully with the proverbial "fire hose" of information that clinical rotations present to the medical student. *High-Yield Obstetrics and Gynecology* is a distillation of the essential information needed by the overwhelmed physician-in-training. This volume is designed to moderate the inevitable indigestion brought on by academic informational hyperphagia.

The outline format and quick-access tables present the key information in a user-friendly format. A recurrent phrase, ***most common,*** is highlighted throughout the book. Special attention should be paid to statements containing this phrase, which frequently form the basis of questions on the United States Medical Licensing Examination (USMLE) Steps 2 and 3. They are summarized in a table "What is the most common . . .?" in the appendix at the back of the book.

The Clinical Situations tables, found at the end of many chapters, emphasize scenarios which call for the Next Step in Management. USMLE 2 and 3 questions commonly end with "What is the next step in management?" Frequently you will be called on to make sequential decisions based on the changing clinical picture. The book text provides the information you need to approach the Clinical Situations. Some new information is provided in the Clinical Pearls of the Clinical Situations, which is not present in the body of the text.

I welcome your suggestions for changes in subsequent editions. Best wishes!

Elmar P. Sakala, M.D., M.A., M.P.H.

Acknowledgments

....

I thank the persevering, inquisitive student physicians whose imaginative questions ensure that my pedagogic arteries will not become prematurely atherosclerotic.

Contents

1

Prenatal Care

I. TERMINOLOGY

A. **Trimester** (a pregnancy is divided into three units of three calendar months)

    1. **First:** from conception to 12 menstrual weeks

    2. **Second:** from 13 to 26 menstrual weeks

    3. **Third:** from 27 to 40 menstrual weeks

B. **Gestational age at pregnancy termination**

    1. **Abortion:** prior to 20 weeks

    2. **Preterm delivery:** between 20 and 37 completed weeks

    3. **Term:** between 38 and 42 menstrual weeks

    4. **Postterm:** after 42 completed weeks

C. **Reproductive history**

    1. **Gravidity:** number of confirmed pregnancies regardless of gestational age or number of fetuses

    2. **Parity:** number of pregnancies terminated on or after 20 weeks

    3. **Abortus:** number of pregnancies terminated before 20 weeks

D. **Developmental periods**

    1. The **embryonic period** begins on the third postconceptional week with the formation of the trilaminar germ disc and extends to the end of the eighth postconceptional week, when the disc has undergone differentiation into all major organ systems.

    2. The **fetal period** begins at the end of organogenesis and extends to birth. It is characterized by growth and maturation of the organ systems.

    3. The **neonatal period** begins at birth and extends to the 28th day of life.

    4. **Infancy** begins at birth and extends to the end of the first year of life.

II. PERINATAL STATISTICS.
Perinatal statistics track outcomes of pregnancies that continue to 20 weeks' gestation or beyond. The standard rates are often used as indices of basic health within a state or the nation (**Table 1–1; Figure 1–1**). Notice the variation between TOTAL and LIVE births in the denominator for the different values.

III. PHYSIOLOGIC CHANGES OF PREGNANCY.
Changes in the anatomy and physiology of the pregnant woman profoundly affect almost all organ systems. Knowledge of these

Table 1–1
Perinatal Statistics

Statistic	Numerator	Denominator
Birth rate	# of live births	1000 total population
Fertility rate	# of live births	1000 females aged 15–45 years
Fetal death rate	# of fetal deaths	1000 TOTAL births
Neonatal death rate	# of newborn deaths	1000 LIVE births
Perinatal death rate	# of fetal + neonatal deaths	1000 TOTAL births
Infant death rate	# of infant deaths	1000 LIVE births
Maternal death rate	# of maternal deaths	100,000 LIVE births

changes is essential to understand many of the medical and obstetrical complications of pregnancy **(Table 1–2).**

IV. **NORMAL LABORATORY FINDINGS IN PREGNANCY.** The reference values for many common laboratory tests are often different for the pregnant woman as compared with the nonpregnant woman. Unless the pregnancy-associated changes in the normal values are understood, interpretation of many laboratory tests in pregnancy may be faulty. Some key laboratory values rise, and others fall **(Table 1–3).**

V. **PRECONCEPTION COUNSELING.** Interventions that could improve the outcome of the planned pregnancy are identified.

   A. Changes in maternal behavior

      1. Women with overt diabetes should **achieve normoglycemia** to prevent fetal anomalies.

      2. Women with increased risk for neural tube defects (NTDs) [previous affected infant, overt diabetes, taking anticonvulsants] should take **folic acid supplements (4 mg/day).** All women of reproductive age should ensure intake of 0.4 mg of folic acid daily.

      3. All women should **avoid teratogenic medications** (see Table 3–2).

      4. All women should **avoid recreational and addictive drugs** (see Table 3–3).

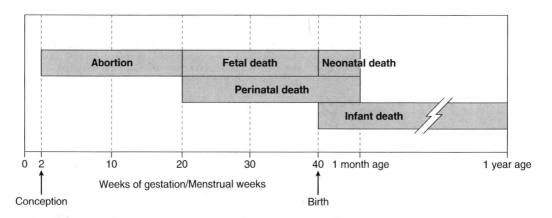

Figure 1–1. Perinatal mortality terminology. (From Sakala EP: *BRS Obstetrics and Gynecology,* 2nd ed. Philadelphia, Lippincott Williams & Wilkins, 2000, p 37.)

Table 1–2
Pregnancy Changes

Organ System	Changes	Result
GI tract	↓ Motility, ↑ water absorption	Reflux esophagitis, constipation
Lungs	↑ Tidal volume, ↑ minute ventilation	Hyperventilation, respiratory alkalosis
Urinary tract	↑ Renal size, ↑ ureteral volume	Urinary stasis, ↑ risk of infections
Heart	↑ Heart rate, ↑ stroke volume	↑ Cardiac output
Arterial	Arterial smooth muscle relaxation	↓ Systolic BP, ↓ diastolic BP
Venous	Venous smooth muscle dilation	Venous stasis, ↑ thrombosis risk
Hematologic	↑ RBC mass (30%), ↑ plasma (50%)	Physiologic dilutional "anemia"
Pituitary	↑ Size, ↑ vascularity	↑ Susceptibility to Sheehan's syndrome

BP = blood pressure   GI = gastrointestinal   RBC = red blood cell

    B. Maternal active immunizations. Women should:

        1. Obtain rubella immunization if they are rubella susceptible.

        2. Obtain hepatitis B virus (HBV) immunization if they are at risk for HBV.

VI. FIRST PRENATAL VISIT

    A. Is the patient pregnant?

        1. Presumptive signs (changes unrelated to the uterus or fetus): amenorrhea, breast tenderness, Chadwick's sign (bluish discoloration of vulva, vagina, and cervix), nausea and vomiting, skin changes

Table 1–3
Changes in Laboratory Values in Pregnancy

	Increased	Unchanged	Decreased
Hepatic	Alkaline phosphatase, all gamma globulins, serum lipids	Liver enzymes (ALT, AST, LDH), bilirubin	Albumin
Renal	GFR, creatinine clearance, glucosuria	Proteinuria	BUN, creatinine, uric acid
Hematologic	WBC, ESR, fibrinogen, clotting factors	Platelet count, PT, PTT, MCV	Hemoglobin, hematocrit
Thyroid	TBG, total T_3, total T_4	Free T_3, free T_4, T_4 index	—
Blood gases	Po_2 pH	Bicarbonate, base deficit	Pco_2
Pancreas	Plasma insulin	—	Fasting glucose
Placental hormones	hPL, hCG, insulinase, estrogens, progesterone	—	—

ALT = alanine transaminase   hPL = human placental lactogen T_3 = triiodothyronine
AST = aspartate transaminase   LDH = lactate dehydrogenase T_4 = thyroxin
BUN = blood urea nitrogen   MCV = mean corpuscular volume T_4 index = free thyroxin index
ESR = erythrocyte sedimentation rate   PT = prothrombin time   TBG = thyroid-binding globulin
GFR = glomerular filtration rate   PTT = partial thromboplastin time   WBC = white blood cell
hCG = human chorionic gonadotropin

2. Probable signs (changes related to the uterus or placenta): uterine enlargement, Hegar's sign (softening between the fundus and cervix), positive β-human chorionic gonadotropin (β-hCG) test, uterine contractions (UCs), palpation of "fetal" parts

3. Definitive signs (changes related to the fetus): ultrasound imaging of the fetus (most specific), auscultation of fetal heart tones (FHTs), x-ray imaging of the fetus, and fetal movements felt by the examiner

B. What is the best estimate of gestational age?

1. Obtain a menstrual history. The last menstrual period (LMP) tends to be reliable if the LMP was definite, the cycle was normal, and the pregnancy was planned.

2. Apply Naegele's rule.
   a. This is a shorthand way of estimating the due date by adding 7 days to the date of the first day of the last normal menstrual period and then counting back 3 months. For example, for an LMP of March 7, 2001, the due date would be January 14, 2002.
   b. Naegele's rule assumes a 14-day preovulatory phase and a 28-day cycle. With shorter cycles, the due date is earlier; with longer cycles, it is later.

3. Obtain a sonogram.
   a. A crown–rump length (CRL) at ≤ 12 weeks is accurate to ± 5 days.
   b. A biparietal diameter (BPD) from 12–18 weeks is accurate to ± 7 days.

C. Are there any risk factors?

1. Medical: diabetes mellitus (DM), hypertension, seizure disorder, cardiac conditions

2. Obstetric: previous perinatal death, fetal anomaly, preterm delivery

3. Family history: inherited diseases, retardation, birth defects, perinatal deaths

4. Lifestyle: alcohol, tobacco, and/or recreational drug use; poor nutrition; eating disorders

5. Psychosocial: abusive relationship, lack of support, poor education

6. Teratogenic exposure: x-rays, toxins, chemicals, medications

D. What prenatal laboratory tests are indicated?

1. Screen for maternal hazards.
   a. Cell profile: anemia
   b. Urinalysis (UA): urinary tract infection (UTI)
   c. Sickle cell prep: sickle cell disease
   d. Tuberculosis (TB) skin test: TB

2. Screen for fetal hazards.
   a. Atypical antibodies: risk of isoimmunization
   b. 1-hour 50-gram glucose load: gestational diabetes
   c. Serology [Venereal Disease Research Laboratory (VDRL) test or rapid plasma reagin (RPR) test]: syphilis
   d. Enzyme-linked immunosorbent assay (ELISA): human immunodeficiency virus (HIV)

3. Identify opportunities for immunization.
   a. Blood Rh status: RhoGAM
   b. Rubella antibodies: postpartum rubella immunization
   c. Hepatitis B surface antigen: neonatal active and passive immunization

4. Screen for fetal anomalies.
   a. Triple marker screen: NTDs, trisomies
   b. Sonogram: gross structural anomalies

E. What patient education is appropriate?

   1. Frequency of subsequent prenatal visits
      a. Every 4 weeks up to 28 weeks
      b. Every 2 weeks from 28–36 weeks
      c. Every 1 week after 36 weeks

   2. Recommended pregnancy weight gain
      a. 30–40 lb if **underweight** (< 90% ideal weight)
      b. 25–30 lb if **average weight** (90%–135% ideal weight)
      c. 15–20 lb if **overweight** (> 135% ideal weight)

   3. Lifestyle recommendations during pregnancy
      a. **Iron** (30 mg of elemental iron/day) and **folate supplementation** (0.4 mg/day) prevents nutritional anemias.
      b. **Alcohol and tobacco intake** of any degree may be hazardous and should be avoided.
      c. **Hyperthermia** (e.g., hot tubs) may be teratogenic during embryogenesis.
      d. **Exercise** can be safely continued at prepregnancy levels.
      e. **Heavy physical work** and **stressful activity** should be avoided.
      f. **Sexual intercourse** is generally safe in the absence of bleeding, ruptured membranes, or preterm labor.

VII. RETURN PRENATAL VISIT

   A. **Are any danger signs present?** Make specific inquiries at each visit **(Table 1–4).** Look for each of the warning signs to identify whether the specific hazard may be present.

   B. **Is there evidence of maternal well-being?** Check for **normal blood pressure (BP)** and **weight gain.**

   1. **Causes of weight loss: dehydration,** hyperemesis, anorexia, bulimia

   2. **Causes of inadequate weight gain: fetal death,** oligohydramnios, intrauterine growth restriction (IUGR), bulimia

   3. **Causes of excessive weight gain: fluid retention,** polyhydramnios, preeclampsia, overeating

   C. **Is there evidence of fetal well-being?** Look for normal fetal movement and FHTs.

Table 1–4
Danger Signs in Pregnancy

Type	Specific Complaint	Condition to Rule Out
Vaginal	Fluid leakage	Rupture of membranes
	Bleeding	Spontaneous abortion, abruptio placentae, placenta previa
Abdominal	Persistent vomiting	Hyperemesis
	Uterine cramping	Preterm labor
	Decreased fetal movement	Fetal jeopardy
	Epigastric pain	Severe preeclampsia
Other	Painful urination	Cystitis, pyelonephritis
	Chills and fever	Pyelonephritis, chorioamnionitis
	Swelling of face and hands	Preeclampsia
	Cerebral disturbances (dizziness, mental confusion, scotomata, new headache)	Severe preeclampsia

D. **Is uterine size appropriate for gestational age?**

    1. **At 12 weeks,** the uterus is palpable at the symphysis pubis.

    2. **At 16 weeks,** the uterus is palpable midway between the pubis and the umbilicus.

    3. **At 20 weeks,** the uterus is palpable at the umbilicus.

    4. **After 20 weeks,** the fundal height measured in centimeters from the pubis should approximate the gestational age in weeks.

VIII. DISCREPANT FUNDAL SIZE (Figure 1–2)

A. **Diagnosis** of discrepant fundal size is made when the fundus measures 3 cm (or more) larger or smaller than expected for the gestational age in weeks.

B. **False discrepancy** (fundal size is appropriate) may be due to:

    1. **Measurement errors:** different examiners, maternal obesity

    2. **Gestational age calculation error:** unsure, irregular, or unusual LMP

C. **True discrepancy** (fundal size is truly too large or too small) may be due to abnormalities of the constituents within the pregnant uterus **(Table 1–5).**

    1. **Fetus:** macrosomia or twins versus IUGR or fetal death

    2. **Amniotic fluid:** The **amniotic fluid index (AFI)** is a sonographic quantification of amniotic fluid volume. The deepest vertical amniotic fluid pocket is measured in each of the four abdominal quadrants. The sum should range between 5 and 25 cm.
        a. **Polyhydramnios** (excessive amniotic fluid): AFI > 25 cm
        b. **Oligohydramnios** (inadequate amniotic fluid): AFI < 5 cm

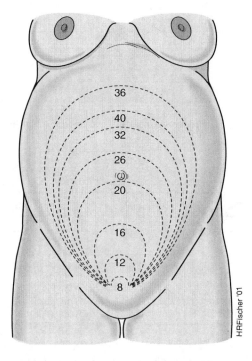

Figure 1–2. Fundal measurement and number of weeks' gestation. (After Scott JR, DiSaia PJ, Hammond CB et al [eds]: *Danforth's Obstetrics and Gynecology*, 6th ed. Philadelphia, JB Lippincott, 1990, p 135.)

Table 1–5
Discrepant Fundal Size

Uterine Contents	Fundal Size	
	Small	**Large**
Fetus	*Too small:* IUGR (symmetric, asymmetric) *Death:* fetal demise	*Too big:* macrosomia (postdates, diabetes, constitutional) *Too many:* multiple gestation (twins, triplets)
Amniotic fluid	*Too little:* oligohydramnios [PROM, fetal urinary tract anomaly, placental insufficiency, or maternal medications (e.g., ACE inhibitors, indomethacin)]	*Too much:* polyhydramnios [decreased fetal swallowing, GI tract obstruction (e.g., tracheoesophageal fistula, duodenal atresia, or twin–twin transfusion)]
Placenta		*Too big:* molar pregnancy (benign or malignant) *Swollen:* placental edema: infection (e.g. syphilis), isoimmunization
Myometrium		*Too much:* leiomyomas, adenomyomas

ACE = angiotension-converting enzyme
GI = gastrointestinal

IUGR = intrauterine growth restriction

PROM = premature rupture of membranes

3. Placenta: hydatidiform mole or edema

4. Uterine wall: leiomyomas, adenomyosis

D. Intrauterine growth restriction (IUGR) is diagnosed if sonographic fetal growth falls below the 10th percentile expected for gestational age. There are two types of IUGR **(Table 1–6).**

1. Symmetric: fetal in origin due to decreased growth potential

2. Asymmetric: placental etiology due to inadequate nutritional substrate availability

Table 1–6
Types of Intrauterine Growth Restriction (IUGR)

	Symmetric	**Asymmetric**
Fetal growth potential	*Decreased*	*Normal*
Time of insult	*Early pregnancy:* usually in first trimester	*Later pregnancy:* usually > 20 weeks
Sonographic findings	*All measurements (BPD, HC, AC, FL)* decreased	*Only one measurement (AC)* decreased (normal BPD, HC, FL)
Etiology	*Fetal problems:* aneuploidy, first trimester infection, severe anomalies	*Placental problems:* hypertension, poor nutrition

AC = abdominal circumference
HC = head circumference

BPD = biparietal diameter

FL = femur length

Clinical Situation 1–1

Basic Case: A 25-year-old multigravida at 28 weeks' gestation who has recently moved to the area comes to the office for her first prenatal visit with you. She brings along records of previous prenatal care. Uterine fundal measurement is not consistent with gestational age.

Patient Snapshot	Intervention	Clinical Pearls
Her **uterus measures 33 cm** from pubis to top of fundus. FHTs are present	Review accuracy of gestational age calculation.	With uterus larger than expected, an **error in dating** must first be ruled out before assuming a true discrepancy in fundal size.
➡ Review of her menstrual history and prenatal records confirms her dates.	Obtain obstetrical sonogram.	With uterus larger than expected, a **sonogram** can rule out twins, macrosomia, polyhydramnios, leiomyoma, or adnexal mass.
➡ The sonogram shows polyhydramnios (with an AFI of 28 cm) and a "double bubble" in the fetal abdomen.	Consider genetic amniocentesis to rule out Down syndrome with duodenal atresia	**Differential diagnosis of polyhydramnios** includes GI tract obstruction (TE fistula, duodenal atresia), ↓ fetal swallowing, and NTD (spina bifida, anencephaly).
Her **uterus measures 24 cm** from pubis to top of fundus. FHTs are present.	Review accuracy of gestational age calculation.	With uterus smaller than expected, an **error in dating** must first be ruled out before assuming a true discrepancy in fundal size.
➡ Review of her menstrual history and prenatal records confirms her dates.	Obtain obstetrical sonogram.	With uterus smaller than expected, a **sonogram** can rule out IUGR or oligohydramnios. Fetal demise is ruled out because FHTs are present.
➡ **Scenario 1** The sonogram shows oligohydramnios (with an AFI of 3 cm). No fetal anomalies are noted.	Watch for cord compression and pulmonary hypoplasia.	**Differential diagnosis of oligohydramnios** includes SPROM, urinary tract anomaly, medications (ACE inhibitors, indomethacin), and placental insufficiency.
➡ **Scenario 2** The sonogram shows that all measurements (BPD, HC, AC, FL) are consistent with 24 weeks. No fetal anomalies are noted	Monitor fetal growth by serial sonograms and tests of fetal well-being (NST, AFI).	**Symmetric IUGR** is indicative of ↓ fetal growth potential due to **early pregnancy insult** (aneuploidy, intrauterine infection, structural anomaly).
➡ **Scenario 3** The sonogram shows that BPD, HC, and FL are 27 weeks but that AC is only 23 weeks. No fetal anomalies are noted.	Monitor fetal growth and fetal well-being (NST, AFI).	**Asymmetric IUGR** is indicative of ↓ placental function due to **late pregnancy insult** [↑ BP, poor nutrition, maternal small-vessel disease (e.g., lupus)].

AC = abdominal circumference
ACE = angiotensin-converting enzyme
AFI = amniotic fluid index
BP = blood pressure
BPD = biparietal diameter

FHT = fetal heart tone
FL = femur length
GI = gastrointestinal
HC = head circumference
IUGR = intrauterine growth restriction

NST = nonstress test
NTD = neural tube defect
SPROM = spontaneous premature rupture of membranes
TE = tracheoesophageal

2

Pregnancy Failure

I. SPONTANEOUS ABORTION

A. Significance. Spontaneous pregnancy loss is common, occurring in at least 15% of known pregnancies, and should be considered whenever bleeding occurs in early pregnancy.

B. First-trimester loss. Early pregnancy loss is largely **fetal** in origin. The *most common* **etiology** is abnormal embryo karyotype **(aneuploidy)**. The *most common* **aneuploidy type** is autosomal trisomy, and the *most common* **single aneuploidy** is monosomy X.

   1. Clinical features. First-trimester loss is usually preceded by vaginal bleeding and cervical dilation, followed by passage of products of conception (POC).

   2. Basis of diagnosis
   a. Extent of vaginal bleeding: spotting, bleeding, or hemorrhage
   b. Ultrasound viability: presence or absence of a gestational sac, fetal pole, cardiac activity
   c. Degree of dilation of the internal cervical os

   3. Clinical entities (Chart 2–1)
   a. Threatened abortion: normal ultrasound with minimal bleeding but without cervical dilation. Rx observation.
   b. Missed abortion: nonviable pregnancy without bleeding or cervical dilation. Rx scheduled D&C.
   c. Inevitable abortion: heavy bleeding and cervical dilation without passage of POC. Rx emergency D&C.
   d. Incomplete abortion: heavy bleeding and cervical dilation present with passage of some but not all POC. Rx emergency D&C.
   e. Completed abortion: passage of all POC with decreased cramping and minimal bleeding with cervical dilation. Rx observation.
   f. Septic abortion: history of nonsterile abortion attempt resulting in uterine infection. Rx admit to hospital for IV multiple agent antibiotics.

C. Second-trimester loss. Later pregnancy loss is usually **maternal** in origin. It is due to uterine anomalies or incompetent cervix.

   1. Clinical features. The clinical history provides a high suspicion of the etiology.
   a. Uterine duplication. Inadequate space in the single uterine horn leads to premature labor with **painful contractions** prior to fetal viability.
   b. Uterine septum and submucous leiomyoma. Inadequate placental vascular supply results in fetal demise.

Early Pregnancy Bleeding
Different diagnoses on the same pathology

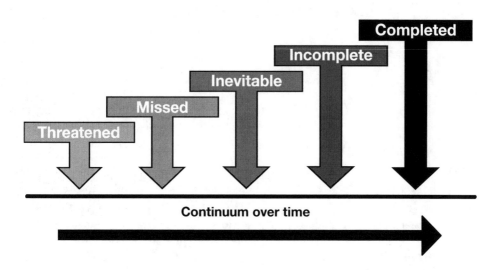

Chart 2–1.

    c. Incompetent cervix. Congenital or acquired cervical weakness leads to passive, **painless cervical dilation,** resulting in delivery of an immature, nonviable fetus.

2. Basis of diagnosis
    a. Hysterosalpingogram (HSG) or **hysteroscopy:** uterine duplication, uterine septum, or submucous leiomyoma
    b. History is diagnostic in women who have experienced a previous pregnancy loss with incompetent cervix after the loss occurred. Risk is assessed based on shortness of cervical length. Diagnosis is based on **vaginal sonography,** revealing a short cervix (< 30 mm long) along with widening of the internal endocervical canal (beaking).

3. Management (Figure 2–1)
    a. Hysteroscopic resection, which removes a thin uterine septum or submucous leiomyoma
    b. Cervical cerclage, which involves a circumferential cervical suture, providing external support to the weak cervix

II. FETAL DEMISE
    A. Overview
        1. Fetal demise is suspected in:
            a. **Early pregnancy** on the basis of **lack of fundal growth**
            b. **Later pregnancy** on the basis of **absence of fetal movements**

        2. Fetal demise is confirmed by **sonographic demonstration of absent cardiac motion.**
    B. Causes
        1. **Idiopathic:** no obvious cause of death even after extensive testing (*most common finding*)

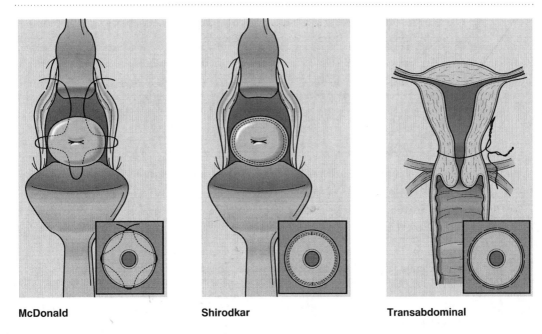

McDonald Shirodkar Transabdominal

Figure 2–1. Management of a patient with an incompetent cervix: McDonald, Shirodkar, and transabdominal methods. (After Scott JR, DiSaia PJ, Hammond CB et al [eds]: *Danforth's Obstetrics and Gynecology*, 6th ed. Philadelphia, JB Lippincott, 1990, p 219.)

2. Placental: severe abruptio placentae; severe infection interfering with oxygen transfer [e.g., *Listeria*, cytomegalovirus (CMV)]

3. Umbilical cord: true knot in the cord; tight nuchal cord

4. Fetal death: lethal aneuploidy; lethal structural anomalies; intrauterine infections; fetal tachyarrhythmias; severe fetal anemia (fetomaternal bleed, severe isoimmunization, parvovirus B19)

5. Antiphospholipid syndrome
 a. Mechanism: attack of the lipid membranes of the fetoplacental unit by **maternal autoantibodies**
 b. Diagnosis: requires any one of the following positive histories AND any one of the following laboratory findings
 c. Positive history: venous thrombosis, pulmonary embolus, or stroke; repetitive pregnancy losses; fetal demise
 d. Laboratory findings: positive anticardiolipin antibodies; positive lupus anticoagulant; prolonged partial thromboplastin time (PTT)
 e. Management: aspirin (80 mg PO every day), heparin (5000 units SQ q12hr)

6. Maternal trauma: direct injury to the fetus; maternal hypotension leading to placental hypoperfusion

7. Diabetes mellitus (DM): uncontrolled hyperglycemia leading to a macrosomic fetus that outgrows placental blood flow and gas exchange, resulting in hypoxia

C. Management

 1. Rule out disseminated intravascular coagulation (DIC). After 4 weeks or more, tissue thromboplastin may be released into the mother's circulation from the deteriorating fetal tissues. **This is a rare life-threatening emergency for which conservative management is never appropriate.**

   2. **Evaluate psychological readiness** for delivery. Delaying intervention may be appropriate to allow initiation of the grief response.

   3. **Select route of pregnancy termination.** Decision-making is related to gestational age, status of the cervix, and necessity for a fetal autopsy.

D. Modes of emptying the uterus

   1. **Dilation and curettage (D&C)** is appropriate for first-trimester demises.

   2. **Dilation and evacuation (D&E)** is appropriate for early second-trimester fetuses where autopsy is not needed.

   3. **Induction of labor** is necessary for any fetuses where autopsy is indicated or later second/third-trimester fetal death. Intravenous (IV) oxytocin or vaginal prostaglandin E_2 (PGE_2) may be used.

III. GESTATIONAL TROPHOBLASTIC DISEASE (GTD)

A. **Definitions.** GTD is a spectrum of neoplasms involving a **proliferative abnormality** of the placenta or trophoblast. These conditions can vary from benign (hydatidiform mole) to malignant (choriocarcinoma).

   1. **Benign GTD,** also known as a **hydatidiform mole,** occurs in two forms **(Chart 2–2).**

Benign GTN - H mole

COMPLETE	INCOMPLETE
Empty egg	**Normal** egg
Paternal X's only	**Maternal & paternal X's**
46, XX (DI ploidy)	**69,** XXY (TRI ploidy)
Fetus **Absent**	Fetus **Non-Viable**
20% ➜ malignancy	**10%** ➜ malignancy

GTN = gestational trophoblastic neoplasm

Chart 2–2.

    a. Complete mole (*most common* form). Dispermic fertilization of an anuclear ovum results in paternally derived normal 46,XX karyotype. Grape-like vesicles are seen without a fetus present. Progression to malignancy is **common** (20%).

    b. Incomplete mole. Dispermic fertilization of a normal ovum results in an abnormal 69,XXY lethal **triploidy** karyotype. No vesicles are present, but a fetus is seen. Progression to malignancy is **uncommon** (5%).

  2. Malignant GTD, known as **gestational trophoblastic tumor,** is classified into good and poor prognosis risk categories **(Chart 2–3).**

    a. Good prognosis (low risk): lower β-human chorionic gonadotropin (β-hCG) titer (< 40,000 mIU/ml) or metastasis to **lungs or pelvis**

    b. Poor prognosis (high risk): higher β-hCG titer (> 40,000 mIU/ml) or metastasis to **brain or liver**

B. Clinical findings

  1. History: bleeding < 16 weeks (*most common* complaint), preeclampsia < 20 weeks, severe hyperemesis, new-onset hyperthyroidism

  2. Examination: vesicles in vagina, absent fetal heart tones (FHTs), uterus larger-than-dates, bilateral theca lutein ovarian cysts

  3. Laboratory finding: excessively high quantitative serum β-hCG titer

  4. Ultrasound: multiple intrauterine echoes without recognizable detail of gestational sac or fetal parts **("snowstorm" pattern)**

C. Management (once diagnosis is confirmed)

  1. Obtain a baseline β-hCG titer. Use to follow declining levels after uterine evacuation.

  2. Obtain a chest radiograph. The *most common* site of metastasis is the **lung.**

  3. Perform a suction D&C. Use oxytocin to contract the uterine venous sinuses and prevent hemorrhage.

Malignant GTN

NON- metastatic	GOOD prognosis	POOR prognosis
Uterus only	**Pelvis** or **lung**	**Brain** or **liver**
100% cure	**> 95%** Cure	**65%** Cure
Single agent chemotherapy		**Multiple** chemo
1 yr. f/u OCs after ß-hCG neg		**5 yr.** f/u on OCs

GTN = gestational trophoblastic neoplasm

Chart 2–3.

4. Provide for contraception. This will prevent confusion of rising β-hCG titers from normal pregnancy with those of recurrent disease.

5. Follow β-hCG titers. Ensure decline to nondetectable levels or identify recurrence. Negative monthly titers are followed up for **1 year** with benign disease or good-prognosis malignancy. **Five-year** follow-up is used with poor-prognosis malignancy.

6. Selectively give chemotherapy. Use only to treat recurrent disease (rising β-hCG titers after D&C) or if histology shows malignant disease. **Methotrexate** or **actinomycin D** are the drugs of choice. A single agent is used with good prognosis disease. Multiple agents are used with poor prognosis disease.

IV. ECTOPIC PREGNANCY

A. Overview

1. Significance. Ectopic pregnancy is the third leading cause of pregnancy-related maternal deaths in the United States.

2. Location. The **most likely sites** of ectopic pregnancy are the oviduct [*most common location* (95%)], the uterine cornu (2%), the abdomen (1%), and ovarian/cervical sites (rare) **[Figure 2–2]**.

3. Risk factors. Intratubal adhesions obstructing the normal passage of the zygote to the uterine cavity are a risk factor; the adhesions may be of either infectious or surgical origin. (However, only 20% of patients with ectopic pregnancy have identifiable risk factors.)

    a. *Most common* **risk factor:** previous salpingitis

    b. Other risk factors: previous ectopic pregnancy, tubal ligation, tubal surgery, intrauterine device (IUD)

B. Clinical findings

1. Symptom triad: amenorrhea, vaginal bleeding, abdominal pain

2. Signs if *unruptured*: cervical motion tenderness, unilateral adnexal tenderness

3. Signs if ruptured (vary depending on degree of hemoperitoneum and hypovolemia): hypotension, tachycardia, peritoneal signs, abdominal guarding

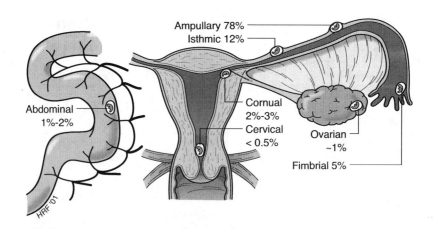

Figure 2–2. Incidence of types of ectopic pregnancy by location. (After Beckmann CR, Ling FW, Barzansky BM et al: *Obstetrics and Gynecology*, 2nd ed. Baltimore, Williams & Wilkins, 1995, p 322.)

   4. Laboratory findings: positive urine or serum β-hCG test (a negative β-hCG value virtually rules out an ectopic pregnancy)

   5. Pelvic sonography: absence of intrauterine gestational sac

   6. Presumptive evidence of ectopic pregnancy: failure to visualize an intrauterine gestational sac with transvaginal sonography when the quantitative **β-hCG titer >1500 mIU/ml**

C. Management is based on whether the pregnancy is early or advanced.

   1. Medical therapy (early unruptured ectopic with serum β-hCG titer < 5,000 mIU) using IM methotrexate, a folic acid antagonist

   2. Surgical therapy (advanced unruptured ectopic with serum β-hCG titer > 5,000 mIU or ruptured ectopic) using laparoscopy, if patient stable, or laparotomy, if patient unstable

   a. Linear salpingostomy (with an unruptured distal tubal ectopic) preserves the oviduct.

   b. Segmental resection (with a ruptured proximal tubal ectopic) allows later tubal reanastomosis.

   c. Salpingectomy (with a destroyed tube or failed tubal ligation) removes the oviduct.

D. Follow-up

   1. RhoGAM is given to prevent Rh isoimmunization if the patient is Rh negative.

   2. Serial β-hCG titers are obtained to ensure complete destruction or removal of viable trophoblast tissue. Obtain these titers if the oviduct is not removed or if methotrexate therapy is used.

Clinical Situation 2–1

Basic Case: A 28-year-old primigravida at 9 weeks' gestation by dates comes to the office.

Patient Snapshot	Intervention	Clinical Pearls
She states she has experienced vaginal spotting for 2 days. Obstetrical ultrasound shows a normal gestational sac, embryo, and cardiac motion.	Use conservative management.	The diagnosis is **threatened abortion.** No therapeutic intervention will change the outcome.
➡ 2 weeks later: She returns to the office stating she has had no bleeding since her last visit. However, a repeat sonogram shows an **empty gestational sac.**	Schedule a suction D&C.	The diagnosis is **embryonic demise** or **missed abortion.** Emptying the uterus by D&C can be scheduled and is not an emergency.
➡ That evening: She comes to the emergency department with bleeding and cramping but has passed no tissue. Pelvic exam shows a **dilated internal cervical os.**	Perform an emergency suction D&C.	The diagnosis is **inevitable abortion.** This pregnancy is doomed. Active intervention minimizes blood loss.
She is bleeding heavily and has passed tissue. Pelvic exam shows a **dilated internal cervical os.** A sonogram shows **retained placental tissue**.	Perform an emergency suction D&C.	The diagnosis is **incomplete abortion.** Act promptly, because bleeding will continue until the uterus is emptied.
She has passed tissue, but bleeding and cramping are now minimal. Pelvic exam shows a dilated internal cervical os, but a sonogram shows **no intrauterine debris**.	Obtain serial β-hCG titers.	The diagnosis is **completed abortion.** Curettage is unnecessary, but because an ectopic pregnancy is possible, follow weekly β-hCG titers until they are negative.
She admits to a lay abortion attempt. Her temperature is 102°F (38.9°C). Her uterus is tender, and pus is coming out of her cervix.	Administer broad-spectrum antibiotics; then perform a gentle suction D&C.	The diagnosis is **septic abortion.** Obtain cultures before starting IV gentamicin and clindamycin. Take care not to perforate this infected uterus.

β-hCG = β-human chorionic gonadotropin   D&C = dilation and curettage   IV = intravenous

Clinical Situation 2–2

Basic Case: A 25-year-old multigravida is being discharged from the hospital after suffering a 17-week spontaneous abortion. She had two previous second-trimester losses.

Patient Snapshot	Intervention	Clinical Pearls
Her previous losses were characterized by 2–3 days of **bleeding** and **cramping** with stillborn fetuses.	Obtain an HSG.	**Müllerian anomalies** can lead to repetitive second-trimester losses due to limited expansion space in the uterus.
➞ **Scenario 1** (3 days later): HSG shows **thick uterine septum** or bicornuate uterus.	Perform laparotomy for corrective surgery.	Also, obtain **IV pyelogram** to rule out urinary tract anomaly, which is ↑ with Müllerian anomaly.
➞ **Scenario 2** (3 days later): HSG shows **thin uterine septum.**	Perform hysteroscopic resection of septum.	**A thin uterine septum** may provide inadequate placental implantation vascular supply.
Her previous losses were characterized by **painless cervical dilation** with rapid delivery of live-born fetuses.	Use cervical cerclage at 14 weeks with next pregnancy.	**Incompetent cervix** treatment is a **cerclage** (a circumferential suture externally supporting the internal os).

HSG = hystersalpingogram   IV = intravenous

Clinical Situation 2–3

Basic Case: A 25-year-old multigravida comes to the outpatient office for a routine prenatal visit.

Patient Snapshot	Intervention	Clinical Pearls
She insists she has felt fetal movements, but a **β-hCG** test is **negative** and a sonogram shows a **nonpregnant uterus.**	Obtain psychiatric evaluation.	**Pseudocyesis** is a conversion reaction in which the patient's intense desire for pregnancy manifests in physical symptoms of pregnancy.
She is 28 weeks by dates and has not felt fetal movement for 2 days. No FHTs are heard.	Obtain obstetrical sonogram to rule out fetal demise.	The diagnostic method of choice with *suspected* **fetal demise** is obstetrical sonogram.
➟ 1 hour later: The sonogram shows a single dysmorphic fetus but no edema. Cardiac activity is absent.	Evaluate psychological readiness for delivery.	For psychological reasons, **delivery** may be **best deferred** to allow the mother to begin the process of **grieving.**
➟ 3 days later: She is emotionally ready for pregnancy termination.	Induce labor with PGE$_2$.	**Labor induction** results in delivery of an intact fetus, allowing autopsy diagnosis of a potentially recurrent syndrome.
➟ After 12 hours of labor, she undergoes a spontaneous vaginal delivery of a dysmorphic stillborn fetus.	Offer options of **seeing** baby, **holding** baby, **naming** baby.	**Grief recovery** is often enhanced when opportunity is given for making the fetal death a reality. Make arrangements for a **fetal autopsy.**
She is 20 weeks by dates with fundus of 16-week size. The sonogram shows fetal demise. Skin edema and abnormal spine angulation are noted.	Rule out DIC.	With unknown duration of demise, **rule out DIC** by obtaining platelet count, fibrinogen, PT, and PTT.
➟ 2 hours later: Lab tests show platelets of 65,000 μl and fibrinogen of 150 mg/dl.	Perform immediate delivery.	The presence of **DIC** constitutes an **obstetrical emergency.** Delivery must not be delayed.
➟ 1 hour later: She is brought to the maternity unit for pregnancy termination.	Perform a D&E.	**D&E** has ↓ maternal mortality than **PGE$_2$** labor induction and is best if a fetal autopsy is not needed.
She is 18 weeks by dates. Routine sonogram shows fetal demise. She has a history of SLE and femoral venous thrombosis.	Rule out **anticardio-lipin antibody syndrome.** Perform D&E.	To rule out this diagnosis, obtain PTT, lupus anticoagulant, anticardiolipin antibodies, antiphospholipid antibodies.
➟ 3 days later: Lab tests show prolonged PTT, elevated anticardio-lipin titer, and elevated antiphos-pholipid antibodies.	In next pregnancy, start treatment in first trimester.	**Anticardiolipin antibody syndrome** is treated with oral low-dose aspirin and subcutaneous heparin.

D&E = dilation and evacuation
DIC = disseminated intravascular coagulopathy
FHT = fetal heart tone

PGE$_2$ = prostaglandin E$_2$
PT = prothrombin time

PTT = partial thromboplastin time
SLE = systemic lupus erythematosus

Clinical Situation 2–4

Basic Case: A 25-year-old multigravida at 16 weeks' gestation comes to the office for a routine prenatal visit, complaining of vaginal bleeding. Her uterus is at the umbilicus, but no FHTs can be heard.

Patient Snapshot	Intervention	Clinical Pearls
She complains of severe nausea and vomiting, stating she has lost 10 pounds over the past month.	Obtain a sonogram to rule out **molar pregnancy.**	Many red flags suggest GTD, including severe hyperemesis, vaginal bleeding, fundus large for dates, and the absence of FHTs.
➤ Even though she has no history of HTN, her BP is 150/90 mm Hg, and her urine dipstick shows 2+ protein.	Obtain a sonogram to rule out **molar pregnancy.**	Molar pregnancy is the only time **preeclampsia** is diagnosed prior to 20 weeks.
➤ 3 hours later: The obstetrical sonogram shows an enlarged uterus without a recognizable gestational sac, fetus, placenta, or amnion.	Schedule a suction D&C after obtaining baseline studies.	The **sonogram** shows the classic "snowstorm" pattern of GTD. Obtain a baseline β-hCG titer and chest radiograph.
➤ **Scenario 1** A suction D&C is performed. The uterine contents histology is consistent with "benign complete mole."	Follow β-hCG titer until negative for **12 months.**	Ensure **effective contraception** for 12 months to avoid confusion of rising β-hCG of normal pregnancy with recurrent molar pregnancy.
➤ **Scenario 2** A suction D&C is performed. The histology is consistent with **malignant GTN** with **good prognostic risk factors.**	Administer **single-agent** chemotherapy and effective contraception.	Methotrexate is administered weekly until β-hCG titers are negative. **Followup** is continued for **12 months.** Remember contraception!
➤ **Scenario 3** A suction D&C is performed. The histology is consistent with **malignant GTD** with **poor prognostic risk factors.**	Administer **multiple-agent** chemotherapy and effective contraception.	Multiple chemotherapy agents are administered weekly until β-hCG titers are negative. **Follow-up** is continued for **5 years.**

BP = blood pressure   FHT = fetal heart tone   GTD = gestational trophoblastic disease
D&C = dilation and curettage   β-hCG = β-human chorionic gonadotropin   HTN = hypertension

Clinical Situation 2–5

Basic Case: A 19-year-old woman comes to the office with unilateral right lower abdominal and pelvic pain.

Patient Snapshot	Intervention	Clinical Pearls
Her LMP was 6 weeks ago, but she is now bleeding. Exam shows she has unilateral right adnexal tenderness and cervical motion tenderness.	Obtain a quantitative β-hCG.	If the quantitative β-hCG is < 5 mIU/ml, any functional trophoblastic villi (including ectopic pregnancy) can be excluded.
➤ 1 hour later: The quantitative β-hCG is 1000 mIU/ml.	Obtain a transvaginal sonogram.	**Pregnancy is confirmed.** A transvaginal sonogram may help differentiate an intrauterine from an ectopic pregnancy.
➤ 2 hours later: The transvaginal sonogram shows no intrauterine gestational sac or pelvic mass.	Repeat the β-hCG transvaginal sonogram in 2–3 days.	With the β-hCG of only 1000 mIU/ml, it is possible this is a normal early intrauterine pregnancy. **The β-hCG should double in 2–3 days.**
➤ 3 days later: The quantitative β-hCG is 2100 mIU/ml. No intrauterine gestational sac is seen on transvaginal sonogram.	Give methotrexate therapy. Follow-up β-hCG titers are needed.	With a quantitative β-hCG ≥ 1500 mIU/ml and no intrauterine gestational sac, **ectopic pregnancy is confirmed.** With early ectopic pregnancy, treatment should be medical.
➤ Her blood type is A negative.	Give RhoGAM.	**Isoimmunization** can occur if Rh-positive RBCs from the placenta enter the patient's circulation.
➤ 1 week later: The quantitative β-hCG titer is rising.	Administer IM methotrexate.	5% of **ectopic** pregnancies removed by linear salpingostomy become **persistent.** IM methotrexate destroys the remaining trophoblastic villi.
Her LMP was 7 weeks ago. Vaginal bleeding began this morning. Now she has acute right lower quadrant pain. Her BP is 70/40 mm Hg, and her heart rate is 150/min.	Emergency exploratory laparotomy.	A **ruptured ectopic pregnancy** is suggested by the triad of amenorrhea, vaginal bleeding, and abdominal pain. Surgical therapy is the only option.

BP = blood pressure
β-hCG = β-human chorionic gonadotropin

IV = intravenous
IM = intramuscular

LMP = last menstrual period
RBC = red blood cell

3

Fetal Medicine

I. PRENATAL DIAGNOSIS seeks to identify anatomic, chromosomal, or medical problems with the fetus prior to delivery.

A. Indications

1. Previous child with anomalies: birth defects, mental retardation, aneuploidy, genetic disease

2. Fetal losses: habitual abortions, fetal demise

3. Previous unexplained neonatal death: death within first month of life

4. Predisposition to anomalies: maternal age $\geq$ 35, overt diabetes

5. Current pregnancy factors: teratogenic exposure, abnormal triple marker screen, abnormal sonogram

B. Methods (Table 3–1)

1. Noninvasive methods are not associated with pregnancy loss.

a. Maternal serum α-fetoprotein (MS-AFP) is a gestational age–specific test. The *most common* cause of abnormal high or low MS-AFP values is **pregnancy dating error.** Low values have only a 20% sensitivity for trisomy 21. Abnormal values should be followed up by sonography and amniocentesis.

b. Triple marker screen is also gestational age–specific. Three blood tests are performed on maternal serum [(MS-AFP, estriol, and β-human chorionic gonadotropin (β-hCG)]. Sensitivity for trisomy 21 is 60%. Abnormal values should be followed up by sonography and amniocentesis.

c. Sonography for fetal anomaly screening is optimally performed between 18 and 20 weeks.

2. Invasive methods are associated with risk of pregnancy loss.

a. Chorionic villus sampling (CVS) is based on the assumption that the fetus and placental villi both arise from the zygote and therefore have the same karyotype.

b. Amniocentesis obtains amniotic fluid and free-floating living fetal skin cells (amniocytes), which can be karyotyped. Single-gene disorder diagnosis can be performed using polymerase chain reaction (PCR) techniques.

c. Percutaneous umbilical blood sampling (PUBS), which has the highest risk of the invasive methods, allows for the widest possible range of fetal testing.

C. Causes of fetal anomalies

1. Polygenic/multifactorial causes (65%). Both genetic and environmental factors are involved. Examples include neural tube defects (NTDs), congenital heart disease, cleft lip, and cleft palate.

Table 3–1
Modes of Prenatal Diagnosis

Weeks	Name	Description	Pregnancy Loss
10–12	Chorionic villus sampling (CVS)	Under sonographic guidance, placental precursors are aspirated either transvaginally or transabdominally for genetic studies.	0.7%
15–20	Maternal serum AFP (MS-AFP)	Maternal serum is tested for levels of AFP (the major fetal serum protein). High values screen for open NTDs, VWDs, and renal anomalies. Placental bleeding and twins give false-positive high values. Low values screen for trisomy 21.	None
15–20	Triple marker screen (X-AFP)	Maternal serum is tested for AFP, estriol, and β-hCG. Trisomy 21 is associated with ↓ AFP, ↓ estriol, and ↑ β-hCG. Trisomy 18 is associated with ↓ levels of all three markers.	None
≥ 15	Amniocentesis	Under sonographic guidance, amniotic fluid is aspirated transabdominally for genetic studies.	0.5%
18–20	Sonography	High-frequency sound waves are used to visualize fetal anatomy screening for structural anomalies.	None
> 20	Percutaneous umbilical blood sampling (PUBS)	Under sonographic guidance, transabdominal umbilical vein funipuncture is performed for assessment/treatment of fetal anemia or genetic studies.	1%–2%

β-hCG = β-human chorionic gonadotropin   NTD = neural tube defect   VWD = ventral wall defect (omphalocele, gastroschisis)

2. **Single-gene disorders (15%) [Figure 3–1].** These are diagnosed by family history and PCR.
   a. **Autosomal dominant disorders.** These gross anatomic lesions have no gender predisposition and have a 50% chance of passage to offspring. Examples are achondroplasia and neurofibromatosis.
   b. **Autosomal recessive disorders.** These biochemical disorders have no gender predisposition and have a 25% chance of passage to offspring. Examples include cystic fibrosis and sickle cell disease.
   c. **Sex-linked recessive disorders.** These disorders are transmitted to offspring on the X chromosome; males are affected and females are only carriers. Examples are Duchenne muscular dystrophy and hemophilia A.
   d. **Sex-linked dominant disorders.** These rare diseases are lethal in male offspring and have no carrier states. An example is hyperammonemia.

3. **Cytogenetic causes (1%).** These are diagnosed by karyotype. The *most common overall aneuploidy* is Turner syndrome (45,X); the *most common trisomy* is trisomy 21.

4. **Teratogenic causes (1%).** External environmental exposures to teratogenic agents within 8 weeks of conception can result in abnormal organogenesis.
   a. **Substances with documented teratogenic effects** are listed in **Table 3–2.** Note the predisposition for IUGR, microcephaly, and craniofacial anomalies.
   b. **Substances that probably have no teratogenic effects** are listed in **Table 3–3.** Although these substances do not cause abnormal organogenesis, they may result in adverse perinatal outcomes.

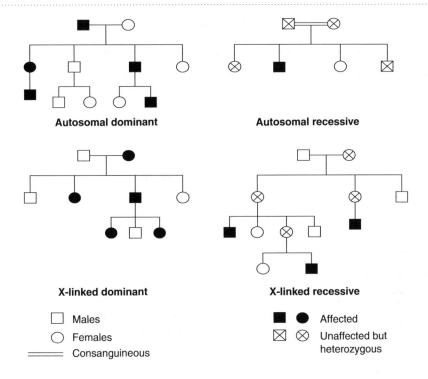

Figure 3–1.   Familial transmission patterns of inheritance. (From Sakala EP: *BRS Obstetrics and Gynecology*, 2nd ed. Philadelphia, Lippincott Williams & Wilkins, 2000, p 52.)

II. ANTEPARTUM FETAL ASSESSMENT

A. Overview

1. **Fetal assessment** seeks to identify fetal compromise early enough to intervene and avoid morbidity and mortality.

2. The *most common* indications for fetal testing are decreased fetal movements, overt diabetes mellitus (DM), postdates pregnancy, chronic hypertension, IUGR, and previous stillbirth.

B. Methods of fetal assessment

1. **Fetal movement counting** involves recording by the mother of the time required for 10 fetal movements. It is not adequate for primary fetal screening in a high-risk population.

2. **Nonstress testing (NST)** is based on an electronic recording of the fetal heart rate (FHR). Heart rate accelerations are seen in a healthy moving fetus at ≥ 30 weeks' gestation. The NST, which is simple to perform, is the *most common* fetal testing method (Figure 3–2).

a. A **reactive NST** requires the presence of FHR **accelerations,** with a rise of ≥ 15 beats/min lasting ≥ 15 seconds, and is reassuring of fetal well-being. **Follow-up** involves repeating the NST weekly or biweekly.

b. A **nonreactive NST** is determined if FHR accelerations are either not seen or, if present, do not meet the criteria (see II B 2 a). This may indicate an acidotic

Table 3–2
Substances With Documented Teratogenic Effects

Substance	Teratogenic Effect
Abused substances	
Alcohol	*Midfacial hypoplasia*, IUGR, microcephaly
Cocaine	*Bowel atresia*, IUGR, microcephaly
Antibiotics	
Streptomycin	*VIII nerve damage*, hearing loss
Kanamycin	*VIII nerve damage*, hearing loss
Tetracycline	*Deciduous teeth discoloration*, tooth enamel hypoplasia
Anticonvulsants	
Carbamazepine	*Fingernail hypoplasia*, IUGR, microcephaly, NTD
Phenytoin	*Nail hypoplasia*, IUGR, microcephaly, craniofacial dysmorphism
Trimethadione	*Facial dysmorphism*, IUGR, microcephaly, cleft lip or palate
Valproic acid	*NTD (spina bifida)*, facial defects
Antivitamins	
Etretinate	Detectable levels may persist for more than 2 years after stopping use (*CNS malformations*, craniofacial dysmorphism, NTD, skeletal abnormalities)
Isotretinoin	*Microtia*, heart and *great vessel defects*, craniofacial dysmorphism
Methotrexate	*CNS malformations*, IUGR, craniofacial dysmorphism
Hormones	
Androgens	*Virilization* of female fetus
DES	*Müllerian duct anomalies*, clear-cell carcinoma of vagina
Heavy metals	
Lead	Miscarriages, stillbirths
Mercury	Cerebral atrophy, microcephaly, blindness
Others	
Coumadin	*Stippled bone epiphyses*, IUGR, nasal hypoplasia
Lithium	*Ebstein's anomaly*, other cardiac disease
Thalidomide	*Phocomelia*, anotia
ACE inhibitors	*Oligohydramnios*, renal tubular dysplasia, neonatal renal failure

ACE = angiotensin-converting enzyme   DES = diethylstilbestrol   NTD = neural tube defect
CNS = central nervous system   IUGR = intrauterine growth restriction

(From Sakala EP: *BRS Obstetrics and Gynecology,* 2nd ed. Philadelphia, Lippincott Williams & Wilkins, 2000, p 55.)

or compromised fetus, but more likely is reflective of a fetus that is asleep, immature, or sedated.

    (1) **Follow-up** involves waking the fetus up with a **vibroacoustic stimulation (VAS)** using an artificial larynx.

    (2) If the NST is still nonreactive after the VAS, a contraction stress test (CST) or biophysical profile (BPP) should be performed.

  3. **Contraction stress testing (CST)** assumes uterine contractions (UCs) decrease intervillous blood flow, resulting in FHR tracing abnormalities in a compromised fetus (see Figure 3–2). If no spontaneous contractions are present, they need to be induced with an intravenous (IV) oxytocin infusion.

    a. A **negative CST** is determined when **no late decelerations** are seen in the presence of three UCs in 10 minutes. This result is reassuring. **Follow-up** involves repeated CST weekly.

Table 3–3
Substances That Have No Probable Teratogenic Effects*

Substance	Specific Agent
Abused substances	Marijuana
Acne drugs	Topical tretinoin
Antiasthma drugs	Beta agonists, prednisone, cromolyn, epinephrine, theophyllin salts
Antibacterials	Penicillins, cephalosporins, clindamycin, erythromycin, metronidazole, nitrofurantoin, sulfa drugs (associated with neonatal jaundice at term)
Anticoagulants	Heparin, enoxarin (low-molecular-weight heparin)
Antidepressants	Tricyclics, monoamine oxidase (MAO) inhibitors, selective serotonin reuptake inhibitors (SSRIs)
Antiemetics	Cyclizine, emetrol, meclizine, chlorpromazine, promethazine
Antifungals	Clotrimazole, miconazole, nystatin, amphotericin B
Antihypertensives	Methyldopa, hydralazine, thiazides (associated with neonatal thrombocytopenia)
Antimalarials	Chloroquine
Antipsychotics	Chlorpromazine
Antituberculosis drugs	Isoniazid, *para*-aminosalicylate, rifampicin, ethambutol
Antivirals	Zidovudine, acyclovir
Cardiovascular drugs	Digoxin, quinidine, propranolol, nifedipine
Contraceptives	Depo-Provera, Norplant, oral contraceptives, spermicides
Minor analgesics	Acetaminophen, salicylates, ibuprofen (may cause oligohydramnios)
Narcotics	Codeine, propoxyphene, oxycodone, meperidine, morphine (all may result in neonatal withdrawal)
Others	Aspartame, caffeine, hair spray

*Although the substances listed do not result in abnormal organogenesis, *they may cause adverse perinatal outcomes.*

(From Sakala EP: *BRS Obstetrics and Gynecology,* 2nd ed. Philadelphia, Lippincott Williams & Wilkins, 2000, p 56.)

b. A **positive CST** is diagnosed when **repetitive late decelerations** are seen with three consecutive UCs. This result is worrisome, particularly if the tracing is also **nonreactive. Follow-up** involves prompt delivery.

4. **Biophysical profile (BPP) testing** adds sonography to electronic fetal monitoring (EFM).
  a. It examines five parameters of fetal well-being.
   (1) **NST reactivity:** presence of accelerations
   (2) **Extremity tone:** extension–flexion
   (3) **Breathing movements:** chest wall movements
   (4) **Gross body movements:** twisting and turning
   (5) **Amniotic fluid volume:** at least one AF vertical pocket ≥ 2 cm
  b. Each parameter is given 2 points if present; if absent, 0 points are given. The highest possible score is 10.
   (1) Scores of 8 or 10 are reassuring. **Follow-up** involves repeating the BPP.
   (2) Scores of 4 or 6 are equivocal. **Follow-up** involves delivery if the gestational age is ≥ 36 weeks **or** repetition in 24 hours if the gestational age is < 36 weeks.
   (3) Scores of 0 or 2 indicate fetal jeopardy. **Follow-up** involves prompt delivery.

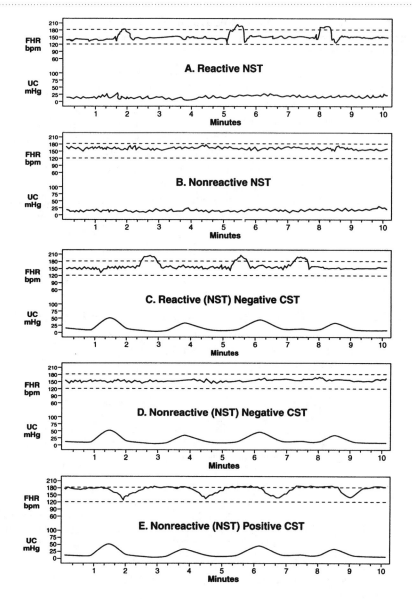

Figure 3–2. Antepartum electronic fetal monitor (EFM) tracings. All EFM tracings should be evaluated for two components: the nonstress test (NST) and the contraction stress test (CST). If a technically adequate fetal heart rate (FHR) tracing is present, the NST component can be assessed as reactive or nonreactive. If three or more uterine contractions (UCs) are present in 10 minutes, the CST component can be assessed as negative or positive. (A) The EFM tracing shows a normal baseline range, and no UCs are present. Thus, only the NST component can be assessed. Because three accelerations are present, the assessment is reactive NST. **This is a reassuring tracing.** (B) The EFM tracing shows a normal baseline range, and no UCs are present. Thus, only the NST component can be assessed. Because no accelerations are present, the assessment is nonreactive NST. **This is not a reassuring tracing,** and the next step should be vibroacoustic fetal stimulation. (C) The EFM tracing shows a normal baseline range, and four UCs are present in 10 minutes. Thus, both the NST and CST components can be assessed. Because three accelerations are present, and no late decelerations are present, the assessment is reactive NST, negative CST. **This is a reassuring tracing.** (D) The EFM tracing shows a normal baseline range, and four UCs are present in 10 minutes. Thus, both the NST and CST components can be assessed. Even though no accelerations can be seen, no late decelerations are present. The assessment is nonreactive NST, negative

III. INTRAPARTUM ELECTRONIC FETAL MONITORING (EFM) seeks to confirm fetal well-being in labor or identify fetal compromise early enough to intervene and avoid morbidity and mortality.

A. Methods

    1. External method. Sonocardiography utilizes an ultrasound transducer positioned on the mother's abdomen to detect fetal cardiac motion. The FHR signal is recorded on a tracing on a moving paper strip.

        a. Advantages. The method can be used any time during pregnancy and does not require cervical dilation or membrane rupture.

        b. Limitations. The quality of the FHR tracing varies with fetal position and may be less precise, especially with maternal obesity.

    2. Internal method. The fetal scalp electrode detects QRS complexes from each fetal cardiac cycle, converting them to an instantaneous heart rate that is recorded on a moving paper strip.

        a. Limitations. Because the cervix must be dilated and membranes must be ruptured, it cannot be used prior to labor.

        b. Advantage. The tracing is extremely precise, providing predictably high-quality recordings.

B. Basic characteristics of electronic fetal monitoring (EFM) tracings

    1. Baseline heart rate: average rate between high and low values

        a. Tachycardia: > 160 beats/min

        b. Normal rate: 110–160 beats/min

        c. Bradycardia: < 110 beats/min

    2. Baseline variability: small, rhythmic heart rate fluctuations

        a. Decreased: ≥ 5 beats/min fluctuations from baseline

        b. Normal range: 5–10 beats/min fluctuations from baseline

        c. Increased: ≥ 11 beats/min fluctuations from baseline

    3. Periodic changes: transitory FHR changes in relation to contractions **(Table 3–4; Figure 3–3; Chart 3–1).**

C. **Interpretation. A reassuring EFM tracing is highly predicative of fetal well-being,** yet most nonreassuring EFM tracings result from nonhypoxemic etiologies. **The *most common* outcome with a nonreassuring EFM strip is a healthy infant.**

    1. Reassuring characteristics

        a. Baseline heart rate: 110–160 beats/min

        b. Baseline variability: 6–10 beats/min

        c. Accelerations: present

        d. Late decelerations: not present

        e. Variable decelerations: no repetitive severe variables (lasts ≥ 60 sec; drops to 60 beats/min below baseline; or drops to ≤ 60 beats/min)

Figure 3–2. (*Continued*)

CST. **This suggests fetal sleep, sedation, or central nervous system (CNS) abnormality.** (*E*) The EFM tracing shows an elevated baseline range, and four UCs are present in 10 minutes. Thus, both the NST and CST components can be assessed. No accelerations can be seen, but repetitive late decelerations are present. The assessment is nonreactive NST, positive CST. **This is highly suggestive of fetal compromise.** (From Sakala EP: *BRS Obstetrics and Gynecology*, 2nd ed. Philadelphia, Lippincott Williams & Wilkins, 2000, p 47.)

Table 3–4
Periodic Changes in Fetal Heart Rate (FHR)

Type of FHR Change	Appearance	Etiology	Prognostic Significance
Accelerations	↑ from baseline heart rate of ≥15 beats/min lasting ≥ 15 seconds	Response to **fetal movement** Mediated by the *sympathetic nervous system*	Always *reassuring*
Early decelerations	Mirror images of contractions	Response to **fetal head compression** *Vagally mediated*	*Benign* (no prognostic significance)
Variable decelerations	Rapid FHR ↓ with rapid increases to baseline with variable shapes	Responses to **umbilical cord compression** *Vagally mediated*	*Benign* if mild or moderate *but worrisome* if severe
Late decelerations	Gradual FHR ↓ with gradual ↑ to baseline after the end of a contraction	Response to **uteroplacental insufficiency**	Always *worrisome*

Mechanism of FHR Decelerations

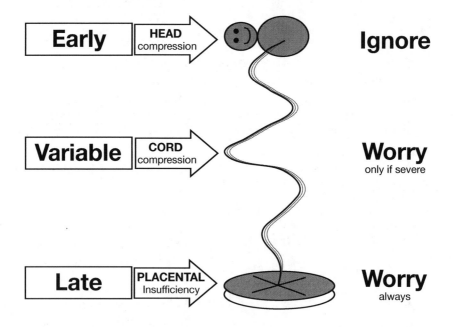

FHR = fetal heart rate

Chart 3–1.

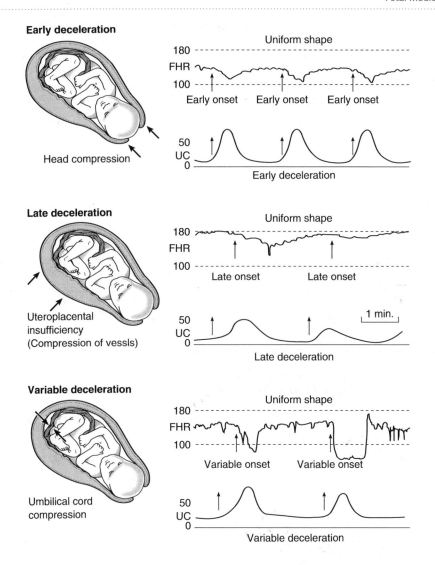

Figure 3–3. Deceleration patterns of the fetal heart rate. (After Hon EH: *An Atlas of Fetal Heart Rate Patterns.* New Haven, CT, Harty Press, 1968.)

2. **Nonreassuring characteristics**
   a. **Baseline heart rate:** tachycardia or bradycardia (without explanation)
   b. **Baseline variability:** minimal or decreased (without explanation)
   c. **Accelerations:** absent
   d. **Late decelerations:** repetitive late decelerations of any degree
   e. **Variable decelerations:** presence of repetitive severe variables

3. The **nonhypoxemic causes** of most nonreassuring EFM tracings include:
   a. **Maternal causes**
      (1) Medications
          (a) **Baseline tachycardia:** scopolamine, atropine, β-adrenergic agonists
          (b) **Baseline bradycardia:** local anesthetics, β-adrenergic blockers

               (c) **Decreased baseline variability:** parasympatholytics, sedatives, tranquilizers

          (2) **Fever:** tachycardia

       b. **Fetal causes**

          (1) **Prematurity:** tachycardia, decreased variability

          (2) **Cardiac arrhythmia:** tachycardia, bradycardia, increased variability

          (3) **Fetal movement:** tachycardia, increased variability

          (4) **Sleep:** decreased variability

       c. **Technical artifacts:** increased variability

   D. **Management of nonreassuring tracings**

      1. **Generic medical interventions to increase fetal oxygenation** are used when EFM tracings are nonreassuring. These interventions vary and include:

       a. **Decreasing uterine activity** by stopping oxytocin

       b. **Correcting maternal hypotension** with a 500-ml bolus of isotonic fluid [e.g., normal saline, Ringer's solution (lactated)]

       c. **Changing maternal position** to relieve possible cord compression

       d. **Administering high-flow oxygen** at 8–10 L/min

      2. **Fetal scalp pH sampling** may be performed in labor after cervical dilation and membrane rupture. This procedure measures capillary blood gases. It is seldom performed in the United States.

       a. A **reassuring** fetal scalp pH is ≥ 7.20.

       b. A **nonreassuring** fetal scalp pH is < 7.20.

      3. **Specific delivery interventions** are utilized when generic interventions do not convert a nonreassuring EFM strip to a reassuring one.

       a. In **Stage 1** of labor: immediate emergency cesarean section

       b. In **Stage 2** of labor: immediate vaginal delivery (using vacuum extractor or forceps if appropriate) or emergency cesarean section

Clinical Situation 3–1

Basic Case: A 39-year-old primigravida at 18 weeks' gestation by dates comes to the Prenatal Diagnostic Center. She undergoes triple marker screening, and the result is abnormal.

Patient Snapshot	Intervention	Clinical Pearls
The X-AFP report shows a positive **HIGH value.**	Obtain a **sonogram** for pregnancy dating.	A **dating error** is the most likely explanation for a high value.
➡ Scenario 1 2 days later: According to the sonogram, gestational age is consistent with 21 weeks, thus explaining the positive **HIGH value.**	No further follow-up is necessary.	Underestimation of actual gestational age gives **false-positive HIGH** triple marker screen **values.**
➡ Scenario 2 2 days later: The sonogram confirms the gestational dating, leaving the positive **HIGH value** unexplained. Sonography shows a positive lemon and banana sign.	Offer **amniocentesis** for **AF-AFP.**	The main concern is a fetal NTD. The sonographic findings are suggestive of spina bifida. The AF sample can be examined for ↑ **AF-AFP.** An ↑ **AF acetylcholinesterase** level confirms an open NTD.
The X-AFP report shows a positive **LOW value.**	Obtain a **sonogram** for pregnancy dating.	The most likely explanation for a low value is a **dating error.**
➡ Scenario 1 2 days later: According to the sonogram, gestational age is consistent with 15 weeks thus explaining the positive **LOW value.**	No further follow-up is necessary.	Overestimation of actual gestational age gives **false-positive LOW** triple marker screen **values.**
➡ Scenario 2 2 days later: The sonogram confirms ths gestational dating, leaving the positive **LOW value** unexplained. Sonography shows thickened nuchal skin fold and short femurs.	Offer **amniocentesis** for **fetal karyotype.**	The main concern is **fetal trisomy 21 or 18.** The fetal karyotype can be obtained by culturing amniocytes floating in the AF.

Clinical Situation 3–2

Patient Snapshot	Intervention	Clinical Pearls
CVS is performed at 11 weeks. The karyotype is reported as 46XX/46XY.	Offer **amniocentesis.**	Placental mosaicism on chorionic tissue can occur with normal fetal karyotype on amniocytes.
A multigravida has delivered an infant with spina bifida. She asks what can she do to prevent recurrence in another pregnancy.	Recommend maternal **folate** supplementation.	**NTD can be prevented by giving folate** (0.4 mg/day for all women; 4 mg/day for those at high risk).

AF = amniotic fluid
AF-AFP = amniotic fluid α-fetoprotein

CVS = chorionic villus sampling
NTD = neural tube defect

X-AFP = triple marker screen

Clinical Situation 3–3

Patient Snapshot	Intervention	Clinical Pearls
A multigravida at 33 weeks reports **decreased fetal movements.**	Perform NST	The **NST** is the **easiest** and most readily available method for confirmation of fetal well-being.
An **NST** of a chronic hypertensive multigravida at 34 weeks is **reactive.**	Repeat the NST weekly.	A **reactive** NST is highly **reassuring** of fetal well-being, with a perinatal mortality rate of 3/1000.
An **NST** of a type 1 diabetic primigravida at 34 weeks is **nonreactive.**	Perform a VAS test.	If stimulation wakes the fetus, resulting in movement, and the NST is reactive, **no further testing** is needed.
➡ 30 minutes later: The **NST** remains persistently **nonreactive** even after VAS.	Perform a BPP or CST.	A **nonreactive NST** does not indicate fetal compromise but **must be followed** by a more specific testing modality (e.g., CST, BPP).
➡ 1 hour later: A **CST** is performed. Oxytocin is infusing, and three UCs are seen in 10 minutes. **No late decelerations** are seen, even though no accelerations are evident.	Repeat the CST in 1 week.	A **negative CST** (even though nonreactive) indicates adequate placental intervillous space blood flow. It is **reassuring** of fetal well-being, with a perinatal mortality rate of 1/1000.
➡ 1 week later: At 35 weeks, a **repeat CST** is performed, and repetitive late decelerations are seen. In addition, no accelerations are seen.	Deliver the infant immediately.	A nonreactive positive CST indicates **serious fetal jeopardy** with high risk of in-utero death.
A **BPP** is performed on a multigravida at 32 weeks with diagnosed IUGR. The NST is reactive. On sonography, the amniotic fluid is adequate. Fetal breathing movements, body twisting, and extremity flexion–extension are seen.	Repeat the BPP weekly.	This BPP score is 10 points, which is the highest score possible. A BPP score of 8 or 10 is highly **reassuring** of fetal well-being, with a perinatal mortality rate of 1/1000.
➡ 1 week later: At 33 weeks, a repeat BPP is performed. The NST is reactive, and on sonography, the amniotic fluid is adequate. However, no fetal breathing movements or gross body motion is seen, even though extremity flexion–extension is noted.	Repeat the BPP in 24 hours.	This BPP score is 6 points, which is equivocal. A BPP score of 4 or 6 is worrisome but not diagnostic of fetal jeopardy. Delivery is deferred due to the early gestational age. At ≥ 36 weeks, delivery would be indicated.

(continued)

Clinical Situation 3–3 (*Continued*)

Patient Snapshot	Intervention	Clinical Pearls
➡ 1 day later at 36 weeks: A **second follow-up BPP** is performed. The NST is now nonreactive, even though on sonography, the amniotic fluid is adequate. No fetal breathing, gross body motion, or extremity flexion–extension are seen.	Deliver the infant immediately.	This BPP score is 2 points, which is ominous. A BPP of 0 or 2 indicates **serious fetal jeopardy** with high risk of in-utero death. Even though this fetus is premature, it should be delivered because the risk of in-utero death is so great.

BPP = biophysical profile   NST = nonstress test   VAS = vibroacoustic stimulation
CST = contraction stress test   UC = uterine contraction

Clinical Situation 3–4

Basic Case: A 23-year-old primigravida is in labor in the maternity unit at term. She is having 45-second duration UCs every 2–3 minutes. Membranes ruptured spontaneously 1 hour ago. Electronic fetal monitoring is in place.

Patient Snapshot	Intervention	Clinical Pearls
The FHR rises 20 beats/min with each UC, returning to baseline after the UC.	Use conservative management.	**Accelerations** are reassuring and associated with fetal movements.
FHR decelerations occur as **mirror images** of the UCs and drop 20 beats/min before returning to baseline after each UC.	Use conservative management.	**Early decelerations** are caused by head compression and do not adversely affect perinatal outcome.
FHR decelerations occur with **rapid drops** of 30 beats/min lasting 30 seconds and are unrelated to UCs with rapid returns to baseline.	Use conservative management.	**Variable decelerations** are caused by umbilical cord compression. They are worrisome only if they are severe.
FHR decelerations occur with **gradual drops** of 30 beats/min, starting after UCs begin with **gradual return to baseline** after UCs are over.	Take generic interventions; perform rapid delivery if no response.	**Late decelerations** are caused by uteroplacental insufficiency and are always worrisome.
The FHR is 170 beats/min with decreased variability and intermittent moderate variable decelerations. **Fetal scalp pH is 7.25.**	Use conservative management.	**Normal fetal scalp pH is $\geq$ 7.20.** This is within the normal range and is reassuring.
The FHR is 170 beats/min with decreased variability and intermittent moderate variable decelerations. **Fetal scalp pH is 7.15.**	Perform immediate delivery.	**Normal fetal scalp pH is $\geq$ 7.20.** This is abnormal, consistent with **fetal acidosis.**

FHR = fetal heart rate   UC = uterine contraction

4

Twin Pregnancy

I. INCIDENCE

  A. Spontaneous ovulation: 1 in 90 births

  B. Ovulation induction: 1 in 10 births (with clomiphene) or 1 in 3 births (with gonadotropins)

II. DIAGNOSIS

  A. Suspicious signs: fundus larger-than-dates, elevated maternal serum α-fetoprotein (MS-AFP) test, excessively high β-human chorionic gonadotropin (β-hCG) titer

  B. Confirmation: multiple fetuses on **obstetrical sonogram**

III. ASSOCIATED RISKS

  A. Fetal risks

    1. Premature delivery (50% of all twins)

    2. Twin–twin transfusion
      a. This condition occurs only with **monochorionic twins** who share a single placenta unequally. The smaller, **donor twin** receives less blood, whereas the larger, **recipient twin** receives more blood.
      b. Diagnosis is made on the basis of **discordance** in **amniotic fluid volume** (oligohydramnios in the smaller twin sac, and polyhydramnios in the larger twin sac).

    3. Umbilical cord problems
      a. Umbilical cord entanglement occurs only with **monoamnionic twins,** who are in a single sac.
      b. Umbilical cord anomalies include velamentous insertion and vasa previa.

    4. Vanishing twin syndrome is seen in early pregnancy when one twin undergoes developmental arrest, leaving only one surviving fetus.

    5. Fetal malformations are most frequent in monoamnionic twins.

  B. Maternal risks

    1. Nutritional anemias (iron and folate deficiency) occur because of the increased requirements of two fetuses.

    2. Risk of **preeclampsia** increases 3-fold.

    3. Risk of **preterm labor** increases 5-fold.

   4. Rate of **cesarean section** increases 5-fold.

C. Obstetrical risks

   1. Risk of **placenta previa** is greater because doubling the placental area increases the risk of lower uterine segment implantation.

   2. Risk of **spontaneous membrane rupture** increases 2-fold.

   3. Risk of **malpresentation** increases 10-fold.

   4. Risk of **postpartum hemorrhage** increases because the overdistended uterus is more likely to develop atony.

IV. CLASSIFICATION OF TWINS (Table 4–1) (Chart 4–1)

A. Zygosity (number of eggs fertilized)

   1. **Perinatal mortality rates** vary in twin pregnancies.
   a. Lowest (12/1000 total births) **in dizygotic twins**
   b. Medium (20/1000 total births) in monozygotic dichorionic twins
   c. Higher (40/1000 total births) in monochorionic diamnionic twins
   d. **Highest** (500/1000 total births) **in monoamnionic twins**

   2. A positive family history increases the chance of monozygotic twins.

B. Chorionicity (number of placentas within the uterus) **[Figure 4–1]**

   1. **Dichorionic twins,** which may be either fraternal or identical, have two placentas and are always diamnionic. Dichorionic twins have the best outcome of twin pregnancies, and the *most common* chorionicity is dichorionic.

Table 4–1
Classification of Twins

By ZYGOSITY	Dizygotic	Monozygotic
Common name	Fraternal	Identical
Number of eggs	Two	One
Prevalence	Two-thirds of twins	One-third of twins

By CHORIONICITY	Dichorionic	Monochorionic
Number of placentas	Two placentas (either separate or fused)	One placenta (shared)
Zygosity	Mono or dizygotic	Only monozygotic
Twin–twin transfusion risk	Low	High
Layers in dividing septum	Four	None or two

By AMNIONICITY	Diamnionic	Monoamnionic
Number of amnions	Two amniotic sacs	One amniotic sac
Zygosity	Mono or dizygotic	Only monozygotic
Chorionicity	Mono or dichorionic	Only monochorionic
Cord entanglement risk	None	High
Layers in dividing septum	Two or four	None

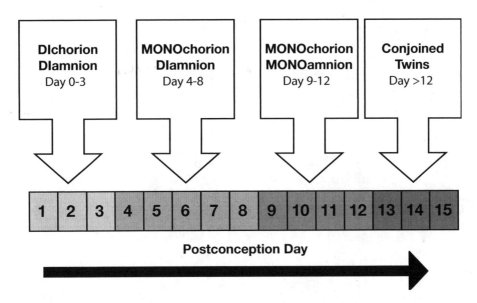

Classification of Identical Twins
by time of splitting

DIchorion DIamnion Day 0-3	**MONOchorion DIamnion** Day 4-8	**MONOchorion MONOamnion** Day 9-12	**Conjoined Twins** Day >12

| 1 | 2 | 3 | 4 | 5 | 6 | 7 | 8 | 9 | 10 | 11 | 12 | 13 | 14 | 15 |

Postconception Day

Chart 4–1.

    2. Monochorionic twins, which are monozygotic and identical, share a single placenta. They can be either diamnionic or monoamnionic and are at risk for **twin–twin transfusion syndrome** diagnosed with discordance of amniotic fluid in the presence of polyhydramnios in one sac and oligohydramnios in the other.

C. Amnionicity (number of amniotic sacs within the uterus) [see Figure 4–1]

    1. Diamnionic twins, which may be either fraternal or identical, have two amniotic sacs with one or two placentas. The *most common* amnionicity is diamnionic.

        a. Monozygotic dichorionic diamnionic twins arise from cleavage at the **morula stage,** which occurs from days 0–3 postconception.

        b. Monochorionic diamnionic twins arise from cleavage at the **blastocyst** stage, which occurs from days 4–8 postconception. They must always be monozygotic.

    2. Monoamnionic twins share a single amniotic sac.

        a. They are always monozygotic, monochorionic, and identical.

        b. They arise from cleavage occurring at the **embryonic disk stage,** which occurs from days 9–12 postconception.

        c. They are at risk for both **twin–twin transfusion syndrome** as well as for **umbilical cord entanglement** and **fetal death.**

        d. Conjoined twins are always monoamnionic and arise from cleavage occurring after day 12 postconception.

V. ANTEPARTUM MANAGEMENT Treatment is based on the risk of twins.

    A. Identify chorionicity and **amnionicity** as early as possible by sonogram.

    B. Ensure adequate maternal nutritional intake (e.g., iron, folate, calories).

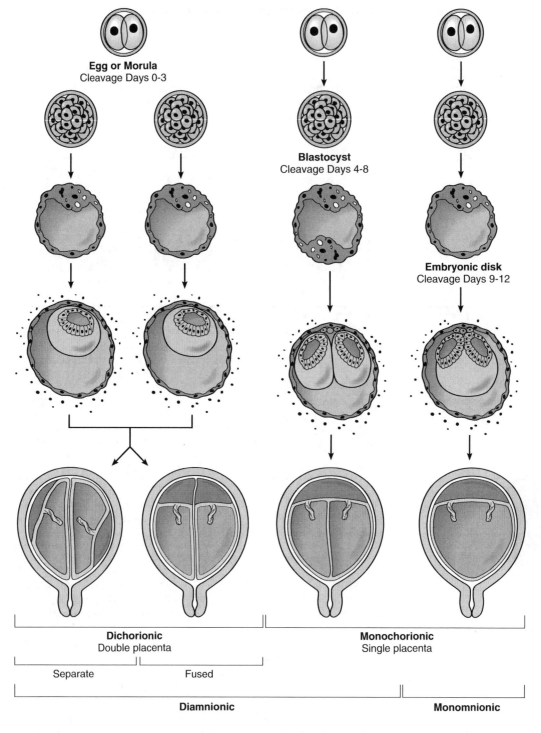

Egg or Morula
Cleavage Days 0-3

Blastocyst
Cleavage Days 4-8

Embryonic disk
Cleavage Days 9-12

Dichorionic
Double placenta

Monochorionic
Single placenta

Separate | Fused

Diamnionic

Monomnionic

Figure 4–1.   Monozygotic twin gestation development. Note the relationship between time of cleavage and the embryonic tissue that divides on the number of chorions and amnions. (After DeCherney AH, Pernoll ML [eds]: *Current Obstetric and Gynecologic Diagnosis & Treatment*, 8th ed. East Norwalk, CT, Appleton & Lange, 1994, p 359.)

C. Educate the mother about premature labor and preeclampsia, and watch for these conditions.

D. Obtain monthly sonograms to monitor fetal growth and well-being.

VI. DELIVERY MANAGEMENT

A. Select the route of delivery based on fetal presentation.

  1. Cephalic-cephalic presentation (*most common*). Vaginal delivery can be anticipated.

  2. Cephalic-breech presentation. Vaginal delivery is possible under certain conditions, but cesarean section is frequently performed.

  3. Breech-cephalic presentation. Cesarean delivery is indicated any time the presentation of the first twin is noncephalic.

B. Watch for postpartum hemorrhage. Give intravenous (IV) oxytocin (10 U/L). If the uterus does not contract well, administer intramuscular (IM) methylergonovine (0.2 mg) and IM carboprost (250 μg).

Clinical Situation 4–1

Patient Snapshot	Intervention	Clinical Pearls
A primigravida at **16 weeks** by good dates has a fundal height at **umbilicus.** She has abnormally elevated levels of MS-AFP and β-hCG.	Schedule a sonogram to rule out multiple gestation.	The combination of fundus larger-than-dates and abnormally elevated levels of MS-AFP and β-hCG suggests **multiple gestation.**
A prenatal **sonogram shows a 7-week pregnancy.** Two embryos are seen in one gestational sac with only **one placenta.**	Schedule a repeat sonogram.	Two embryos in one sac suggest **monoamnionic twins. It is crucial to rule out conjoined twins.**
Two fetuses are apparent on informal sonogram at 14 weeks.	Schedule a formal sonogram. Give iron and folate.	Pregnancy risk with twins is determined by identifying **chorionicity** and **amnionicity** as early as possible.
A primigravida is at **28 weeks with confirmed twins,** one male and one female.	Serially monitor BP and fetal growth, and watch for preterm labor.	Different genders can occur only in a **dizygotic pregnancy.** All twins pose an increased risk for preeclampsia, IUGR, and preterm labor.
A primigravida is at **28 weeks with confirmed monochorionic, diamnionic twins.**	Monitor closely for fetal growth and amniotic fluid volumes.	**Monochorionic twins** require serial sonograms, looking for evidence of **twin–twin transfusion.**
A primigravida is at **28 weeks with confirmed monochorionic, monoamnionic twins.**	Hospitalize, watching for variable decelerations.	**Monoamnionic twins are at risk for umbilical cord entanglement** (and fetal demise) as well as twin–twin transfusion.

BP = blood pressure   IUGR = intrauterine growth restriction   MS-AFP = maternal serum α-fetoprotein

Clinical Situation 4–2

Basic Case: A multigravida pregnant with twins at 36 weeks is in the maternity suite.

Patient Snapshot	Intervention	Clinical Pearls
She is in labor with a **cephalic-cephalic presentation.**	Perform vaginal delivery.	With both twins in cephalic presentation, **vaginal delivery** provides as good a perinatal outcome as CS with fewer maternal risks.
She is in labor with a **cephalic-breech presentation.**	Perform vaginal delivery or emergency CS.	Under certain conditions, the breech second twin can be delivered vaginally. Otherwise, CS is best.
She is in labor with a **breech-breech presentation.**	Perform emergency CS.	Whenever the first twin is non-cephalic in presentation, **CS** is safer for the infants.
The **placentas have just been delivered after a vaginal delivery of twin neonates.**	Give IV oxytocin; have IM methyl-ergonovine and IM dinoprost ready.	**Postpartum hemorrhage** is common after a distended uterus does not contract well after delivery.

CS = cesarean section

5

Third-Trimester Bleeding

I. OVERVIEW

A. Third-trimester bleeding is potentially life-threatening to both the mother and the fetus and must be taken seriously.

B. The first priority is to assess vital signs of the mother (pulse and blood pressure) and to evaluate fetal status. If either the mother or the fetus is unstable, the mother should be stabilized and then the fetus should be delivered immediately by the most appropriate route.

C. **Never perform a speculum examination or a digital examination until placenta previa has been ruled out by obstetrical ultrasound.** This action could trigger a massive hemorrhage.

II. CAUSES

A. **Nonobstetric.** Patients usually present with vaginal spotting from a cervical polyp, vaginal lesion, or varicosity. Diagnosis is by speculum examination.

B. **Obstetric.** Bleeding may or may not be painful. Causes include placenta previa, vasa previa, abruptio placentae, and uterine rupture.

III. PAINLESS BLEEDING (Table 5–1) is characteristic of placenta previa and vasa previa.

A. **Placenta previa** is the *most common* cause of **painless** third-trimester bleeding (Figure 5–1).

    1. This condition is diagnosed when the location of placental implanted is abnormal—in the **lower uterine segment.** Seen frequently on second-trimester sonograms, it is less apparent at term.

    2. The mechanism of placenta previa decreasing with gestational age involves **"placental migration,"** which results from progressive placental atrophy in the poorly vascularized lower uterine placenta and hypertrophy of the better perfused upper fundal placenta.

    3. **Maternal blood** is the source of the bleeding.

B. **Vasa previa** is rare.

    1. This condition occurs as the result of rupture of the fetal vessels that cross the membranes covering the cervix. These abnormal vessels connect the main placenta to a succenturiate (accessory) lobe or to a velamentous umbilical cord.

    2. Diagnosis is seldom made <u>until **rupture of membranes**</u> results in acute **vaginal bleeding** and **fetal bradycardia.**

Table 5–1
Etiology of Painless Third-Trimester Bleeding

Characteristics	Placenta Previa	Vasa Previa
Frequency	0.5% of deliveries at term	Rare
Mechanism	Avulsion of anchoring villi of a *low-implanted placenta,* with stretching of the lower uterine segment	*Rupture of fetal vessels* crossing the placental membranes that lie over the cervix
Risk factors	Multiple gestation, previous placenta previa, multiparity, advanced maternal age	Multiple gestation, velamentous cord insertion, accessory placental lobe
Types	*Complete:* covers internal cervical os *Partial:* partially over interval cervical os *Low-lying:* close to internal cervical os	—
Management	*Dependent* on gestational age and stability of mother and fetus	Immediate *emergency cesarean section*

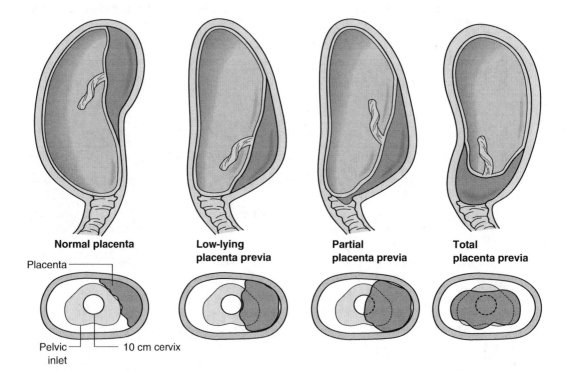

Figure 5–1.   Diagnostic classification of placenta previa: (*A*) Normal, (*B*) low-lying, (*C*) partial, and (*D*) total. (After DeCherney AH, Pernoll ML [eds]: *Current Obstetrics & Gynecologic Diagnosis & Treatment,* 8th ed. East Norwalk, CT, Appleton & Lange, 1994, p 404.)

Table 5–2
Etiology of Painful Third-Trimester Bleeding

Characteristics	Abruptio Placentae	Uterine Rupture
Frequency	1% of deliveries	Rare
Mechanism	Hemorrhage into decidua basalis behind *normally implanted placenta*	Full-thickness laceration of myometrial wall with or without previous uterine scar
Risk factors	Hypertension, trauma, cocaine, PROM, previous abruptio placentae	Previous uterine scar, excessive oxytocin, overdistended uterus
Types	*Overt:* external vaginal bleeding *Concealed:* bleeding remaining retro-placental and only internal	*Complete:* communication of uterine laceration with peritoneal cavity *Incomplete:* peritoneum remaining intact
Management	*Dependent* on gestational age and stability of mother and fetus	Immediate *emergency cesarean section*

PROM = premature rupture of membranes

3. Fetal blood is the source of the bleeding. Fetal exsanguination will occur if delivery is not immediate.

IV. PAINFUL BLEEDING (Table 5–2) is characteristic of abruptio placentae and uterine rupture.

   A. Abruptio placentae is the *most common* cause of all third-trimester bleeding, the *most common* cause of painful third-trimester bleeding, and the *most common* obstetric cause of disseminated intravascular coagulation (DIC) [**Figure 5–2**].

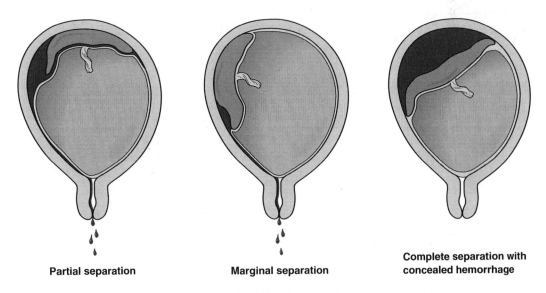

Partial separation   **Marginal separation**   **Complete separation with concealed hemorrhage**

Figure 5–2. Diagnostic classification of types of abruptio placentae: partial, marginal, and complete separation with concealed hemorrhage. (After Scott JR, DiSaia PJ, Hammond CB et al [eds]: *Danforth's Obstetrics and Gynecology*, 6th ed. Philadelphia, JB Lippincott, 1990, p 560.)

1. This condition is diagnosed with painful vaginal bleeding in the presence of a normally implanted upper uterine placenta.

2. The risk of complications varies with the degree of abruption; as separation of the placenta progresses from mild to complete, the risk increases.

B. **Uterine rupture** results in 50% of fetal deaths and 5% of maternal deaths.

1. This diagnosis should be considered with heavy bleeding in the presence of a contracted uterus.

2. It must be distinguished from **uterine dehiscence,** which is a gradual, asymptomatic separation of a uterine scar without bleeding.

V. MANAGEMENT

A. Patient stabilization is the next immediate step.

B. Immediate cesarean section is essential as soon as diagnosis of **vasa previa** or **uterine rupture** is made.

C. A vaginal examination should never be performed until placenta previa has been ruled out by sonographic localizing of placental implantation.

D. Selection of **conservative or aggressive management** (emergency cesarean section) with abruptio placentae and placental previa depends on:

1. Presence or absence of **maternal stability**

2. Presence or absence of **fetal stability**

3. Mature or immature **gestational age**

Clinical Situation 5–1

Basic Case: A 25-year-old primigravida at 32 weeks' gestation comes to the maternity unit with pain-less bright-red vaginal bleeding.

Patient Snapshot	Intervention	Clinical Pearls
The patient's vital signs are stable: BP, 120/75 mm Hg; heart rate, 95 beats/min; respirations, 18/min. The fetal monitor shows a reactive tracing.	Obtain sonogram for placental localization.	The first priority is to stabilize the patient. The sonogram differentiates abruptio placentae from placenta previa. **Avoid digital cervical exam.**
➤ 1 hour later: Sonography shows the fetus in transverse lie, with the placenta completely over the internal cervical os.	Hospitalize with conservative management.	With placenta previa remote from term, **manage conservatively,** hoping to prolong the pregnancy for fetal benefit.
➤ **Scenario 1** After 2 weeks of hospitalization for placenta previa: She is now **bleeding heavily** again, with FHR showing bradycardia at 90 beats/min.	Perform an immediate cesarean delivery.	With placenta previa and an **unstable mother or fetus,** regardless of gestational age, **delivery without delay** is essential.
➤ **Scenario 2** After 5 weeks of hospitalization for placenta previa: Fetus is in transverse lie. Amniocentesis shows an **L/S** ratio of **3.1.**	Schedule a CS.	When **fetal lung maturity** is confirmed with total placenta previa, there is no benefit to either the mother or fetus in prolonging the pregnancy.
AROM has just been per-formed in active labor. Immediate vaginal **bleeding** and **fetal brady-cardia** occur.	Perform a "crash" CS.	This triad is classic for a bleeding **vasa previa.** The fetus will die in minutes if not delivered immediately.

AROM = artificial rupture of membranes FHR = fetal heart rate   L/S = lecithin/sphingomyelin

Clinical Situation 5–2

Basic Case: A 25-year-old multigravida at 32 weeks comes to the maternity unit with painful bright-red vaginal bleeding. A sonogram at 19 weeks showed a fundal placenta without placenta previa.

Patient Snapshot	Intervention	Clinical Pearls
Initially, she had vaginal bleeding and painful UCs, but now bleeding and cramping have stopped. The mother's vital signs and FHTs are stable.	Hospitalize with conservative management.	This scenario presents as a self-limited **mild abruption** that has stabilized. With a premature but stable fetus, **conservative management** is appropriate.
She has constant uterine pain, but is now 10 cm dilated, +2 station. FHR is 145 beats/min without decelerations.	Allow vaginal delivery.	The scenario is consistent with **abruptio placentae.** Because the mother and fetus are stable and rapid delivery is expected, **conservative management** is appropriate.
She has constant uterine pain but is only 2 cm dilated. Her BP is **80/40 mm Hg** and heart rate is 130 beats/min. FHR reveals **bradycardia** (70 beats/min).	Perform immediate CS.	An **unstable abruptio placentae** is an obstetrical emergency. After the mother has been stabilized, the **fetus should be delivered promptly.**
She had a previous CS through a **classical uterine incision.** Her BP is **70/45 mm Hg** and heart rate is 140 beats/min. FHR is unobtainable. Abdominal exam shows rigidity and guarding.	Perform immediate exploratory laparotomy.	This scenario presents as an acute **uterine rupture** with massive intraperitoneal bleeding. The urgent need is to stop the bleeding and save the fetus if possible.

BP = blood pressure   FHR = fetal heart rate   UC = uterine contraction
CS = cesarean section   FHT = fetal heart tone

6

Isoimmunization

I. DEFINITION

A. Isoimmunization occurs when a woman produces antibodies against foreign red blood cell (RBC) antigens in the maternal circulation. These antibodies have the potential to cross the placenta and hemolyze fetal RBC.

B. Foreign RBCs include not only those with the rhesus antigens (C, c, D, E, e) but also those with Kell, Kidd, and Duffy antigens. The *most common* isoimmunization antigen is D.

II. PATHOPHYSIOLOGY

A. The lymphocytes of a pregnant woman are exposed to foreign RBC antigens either from a fetomaternal bleed during a previous pregnancy or blood transfusion. The activated maternal lymphocytes produce atypical IgG antibodies that can cross the placenta to attack antigen-positive fetal RBCs.

B. If the maternal antibody titer is high, and enough antibodies cross the placenta, they produce fetal RBC hemolysis, resulting in fetal anemia and hydrops, and perhaps even death.

III. CLINICAL APPROACH

A. Prevent Rho (D) isoimmunization.

   1. Identify at-risk pregnancies, and then administer RhoGAM to the mother. The RhoGAM binds to and hemolyzes any D-positive RBCs in her circulation.

   2. Indications for RhoGAM include at 28 weeks' gestation (*most common* use); after delivery of Rh-positive neonates; and after amniocentesis, ectopic pregnancy, first-trimester dilation and curettage (D&C), and third-trimester bleeding.

   3. Give RhoGAM 300 μg intramuscularly (IM) within 72 hours of the fetomaternal bleed.

B. Identify if the fetus is at risk for RBC hemolysis and anemia. Fetal risk is present only if all the following are present:

   1. The mother is RBC antigen–negative and the fetus is RBC antigen–positive. (The fetus can only be RBC antigen–positive if the father is RBC antigen–positive.)

   2. The mother has atypical antibodies against the fetal RBC antigen.

   3. The fetal RBC antigen is associated with hemolytic disease of the newborn (HDN).

   4. The titer of atypical antibodies in the mother's circulation is $\geq$ 1:8.

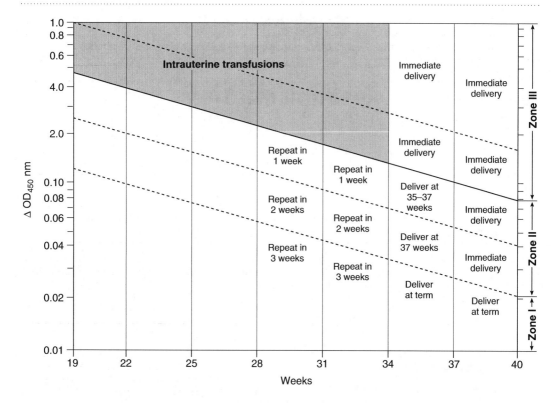

Figure 6–1. Liley graph for isoimmunization management. (After Hacker NF, Moore JG [eds]: *Essentials of Obstetrics and Gynecology*, 2nd ed. Philadelphia, WB Saunders, 1992, p 303.)

C. Identify evidence of fetal anemia.

    1. Assess anemia **indirectly** by analyzing amniotic fluid (obtained by amniocentesis) for bilirubin level (change in optical density at 450 nm [ΔOD_{450}]). The ΔOD_{450} value is then plotted on a Liley graph in zone I, II, or III to assess the risk of fetal anemia **(Figure 6–1).**

    2. Assess anemia **directly** by performing percutaneous umbilical blood sampling (PUBS).

    3. Assess anemia **indirectly** by ultrasound measurement of fetal middle cerebral artery velocity. Also look for fetal hydropic changes.

D. Determine whether the anemia is severe enough to require intervention.

    1. Criteria for intervention: amniotic fluid bilirubin in Liley zone III, fetal hematocrit ≤ 25%

    2. Interventions
        a. Delivery if gestational age ≥ 34 weeks
        b. Intrauterine transfusion if gestational age < 34 weeks

Clinical Situation 6–1

Basic Case: A 21-year-old primigravida has a **negative atypical antibody screen (AAS).**

Patient Snapshot	Intervention	Clinical Pearls
Gestational age is 16 weeks, her blood type is **O-negative,** and she has just undergone a genetic amniocentesis.	Give RhoGAM now.	Fetal RBCs could have entered the mother's circulation during the amniocentesis, placing her at risk for Rh (D) isoimmunization. Prophylactic RhoGAM can reduce the risk.
Gestational age is 28 weeks and her blood type is **O-positive.**	No further workup is indicated.	If her blood is O-positive, the mother has no risk factors for Rh (D) isoimmunization.
Gestational age is 28 weeks and her blood type is **O-negative.**	Give RhoGAM now.	Because the mother is O-negative, she is at risk for Rh (D) isoimmunization. Prophylactic RhoGAM can reduce the risk.
She is 1-day postpartum after a term spontaneous vaginal delivery of an **Rh-positive** infant. Her blood type is **O-negative.**	Give RhoGAM now.	RhoGAM 300 μg IM given within 72 hours attacks any fetal RBCs in the mother's circulation, thus preventing lymphocyte activation.
She is 1-day postpartum after a term spontaneous vaginal delivery of an **Rh-negative** infant. Her blood type is **O-negative.**	No further workup is indicated.	Because both the mother and infant are Rh-negative, no risk of maternal isoimmunization exists, and thus no RhoGAM is indicated.
She is 1-day postpartum after a 32-week emergency CS delivery performed because of abruptio placentae. The infant is **Rh-positive.** Her blood type is **O-negative.**	Estimate the number of fetal RBCs in the mother's blood.	A **Kleihauer-Betke** test estimates the fetal blood volume in the maternal circulation. Administer RhoGAM 300 μg IM for each 15 ml of fetal RBCs.

CS = cesarean section   RhoGAM = Rh (D) immune globulin   RBC = red blood cell

Clinical Situation 6–2

Basic Case: A 21-year-old primigravida at 28 weeks' gestation presents with a **positive AAS.**

Patient Snapshot	Intervention	Clinical Pearls
Her blood type is **O-positive.**	Type the **atypical antibody.**	If the atypical antibody is **not associated with HDN,** there is no fetal risk.
Her blood type is **O-negative.**	Type the **atypical antibody.**	The atypical antibody cannot be assumed to be anti-D. Its **identity must be determined** to see if it is associated with HDN.
➤ 3 days later: AAS typing shows **anti-Kidd antibodies associated with HDN.**	Determine the **Kidd antigen status** of the **father's RBCs.**	If the **father's RBCs are Kidd antigen–negative,** there is **no fetal risk** of hemolysis and anemia, regardless of how high the antibody titer is.
➤ 4 days later: The father's RBCs are **Kidd antigen–positive.**	Determine the **anti-Kidd antibody titer** of the mother.	**Fetal risk** of hemolysis and anemia is likely only when atypical antibody concentrations are high (> **1:8**).
➤ 5 days later: The mother's **anti-Kidd titer** is **1:4.**	**Repeat atypical antibody titer monthly.**	With a low titer of 1:4, there is **low risk** that enough antibodies will cross the placenta to cause fetal anemia.
The father's RBCs are **Kidd antigen–negative.**	No further workup is indicated.	Because **both the mother and father are Kidd antigen–negative,** the fetus must also be Kidd antigen–negative and is therefore at **no risk for HDN.**

AAS = atypical antibody screen   HDN = hemolytic disease of the newborn   RBC = red blood cell

Clinical Situation 6–3

Basic Case: A 21-year-old primigravida at 28 weeks' gestation presents with **an anti-Kidd titer > 1:8.** The father of the pregnancy is Kidd antigen–positive.

Patient Snapshot	Intervention	Clinical Pearls
The mother's **anti-Kidd titer** is **1:32.**	Perform either amniocentesis for AF bilirubin level or PUBS for fetal hematocrit.	With a high titer of 1:32, there is **significant risk of fetal hemolysis.** The AF bilirubin is an indirect indication of the degree of fetal RBC hemolysis. The fetal hematocrit directly assesses fetal anemia.
➡ 2 days later: an amniocentesis reveals the AF bilirubin (ΔOD_{450}) in **Liley zone I.**	**Repeat amniocentesis** in 3 weeks.	In zone I, this fetus has either **no anemia** or **only mild anemia.** Conservative management has less risk than intervention.
➡ 3 weeks later: a repeat amniocentesis reveals the AF bilirubin (ΔOD_{450}) in lower **Liley zone II.**	**Repeat amniocentesis** in 2 weeks.	In lower zone II, this fetus probably has **mild-to-moderate anemia.** However, conservative management still has less risk than intervention.
The fetal hematocrit by **PUBS** is **35%.**	**Repeat PUBS** in 3 weeks.	This fetus has only **mild anemia.** Conservative management has less risk than intervention.

AF = amniotic fluid   PUBS = percutaneous umbilical blood sampling   RBC = red blood cell

Clinical Situation 6–4

Basic Case: A 21-year-old primigravida has an **anti-Kidd titer of 1:64.**

Patient Snapshot	Intervention	Clinical Pearls
The gestational age is **28 weeks.** Fetal Hct by **PUBS** is **15%** or AF bilirubin (ΔOD_{450}) is in **Liley zone III.**	**Intervene** with an **intrauterine transfusion.**	With low Hct or high AF bilirubin, this fetus probaly has **severe life-threatening anemia,** so intervention is necessary. Intrauterine transfusion is less risky than premature delivery.
The gestational age is **35 weeks.** Fetal Hct by **PUBS** is **15%** or AF bilirubin (ΔOD_{450}) is in **Liley zone III.**	**Deliver promptly.**	With low Hct or high AF bilirubin, this fetus probably has **severe life-threatening anemia,** so intervention is necessary. Delivery after 34 weeks is less risky than intrauterine transfusion.

AF = amniotic fluid   Hct = hematocrit   PUBS = percutaneous umbilical blood sampling

7

Hypertension in Pregnancy

I. OVERVIEW

A. Definition. Diagnosis of hypertension requires **sustained** blood pressure (BP) elevation of $\geq 140/90$ at bed rest on two occasions at least 6 hours apart.

B. Prevalence. Hypertension occurs in up to 10% of all pregnancies.

II. CLASSIFICATION according to the NIH Working Group Report on High Blood Pressure in Pregnancy (2000)

A. Chronic hypertension (HTN) is defined as hypertension present prior to the pregnancy or that is diagnosed before 20 weeks' gestation. Proteinuria may or may not be present. Perinatal outcome is usually good if the pregnancy is not complicated by superimposed preeclampsia or IUGR **(Chart 7–1)**.

    1. Good outcome. Perinatal outcome is usually good if the hypertension is mild (BP ≤ 180 mm Hg systolic or ≤ 110 mm Hg diastolic), there is no evidence of end-organ damage, and fetal growth is appropriate.

    2. Poor outcome. Pregnancy complications are increased with moderate hypertension (BP ≥ 180 mm Hg systolic or ≥ 110 mm Hg diastolic) or significant end-organ damage (serum creatinine > 1.4 mg/dL, hypertensive retinopathy, left ventricular hypertrophy).

    3. Worst outcome. Pregnancy complications are the highest with out-of-control hypertension (BP ≥ 210 mm Hg systolic or ≥ 120 mm Hg diastolic).

B. Preeclampsia-eclampsia is a pregnancy-specific syndrome that usually occurs after 20 weeks' gestation **(Table 7–1)**. Edema is no longer a criteria for preeclampsia. *The risk of later developing chronic hypertension is <u>not</u> increased.*

    1. Mild preeclampsia is defined as hypertension developing during the pregnancy accompanied by proteinuria (≥ 300 mg in 24 hours or $\geq 1+$ on dipstick) with no evidence of UTI. Headache, epigastric pain, and visual changes are absent. Hemoconcentration ($\uparrow$ hemoglobin, $\uparrow$ hematocrit, $\uparrow$ serum uric acid) is frequently seen.

    2. Severe preeclampsia is less common. It can be diagnosed on the basis of severe hypertension (≥ 160 mm Hg systolic or ≥ 110 mm Hg diastolic) or severe proteinuria (≥ 2.0 g in 24 hrs or $2+$ or $3+$ on dipstick). It can also be diagnosed in the presence of only mild hypertension and proteinuria if any of the following are present:
        a. Laboratory findings: elevated serum creatinine (> 1.2 mg/dL); thrombocytopenia (platelet count $< 100,000$ cells/mm3); hemolysis ($\uparrow$ LDH); $\uparrow$ liver enzymes (ALT, AST).

Chronic HTN
Pregnancy Prognosis

GOOD prognosis	**BP 140/90 to 179/109** No end-organ damage

POOR prognosis	**KIDNEYS:** renal disease Creatinine > 1.4 mg/dL
	EYES: retinopathy Hemorrhages, exudates, narrowing
	HEART: LVH Prolonged BP > 180/110

WORST prognosis	**Uncontrolled HTN** Chronic HTN + superimposed PIH

HTN = hypertension LVH = left ventricular hypertrophy PIH = pregnancy-induced hypertension

Chart 7–1.

    b. Symptoms: epigastric pain, persistent headache, visual disturbances

    3. Eclampsia is the occurrence in a woman with preeclampsia of seizures that cannot be attributed to other causes.

C. Preeclampsia superimposed on chronic hypertension is diagnosed in women with chronic hypertension and no proteinuria who experience new-onset proteinuria or women with chronic hypertension AND proteinuria who experience sudden increase in proteinuria, sudden increase in BP, thrombocytopenia, or elevation of liver enzymes.

D. Gestational hypertension is a non-specific diagnosis that is made in the presence of hypertension after 20 weeks' gestation WITHOUT proteinuria. It may represent impending preeclampsia prior to development of proteinuria or new onset of chronic hypertension during the pregnancy. This diagnosis is used during pregnancy only until a more specific diagnosis can be diagnosed postpartum.

E. Transient hypertension is a retrospective postpartum diagnosis made after gestational hypertension returns to normal levels following delivery. *The risk of subsequent development of chronic hypertension is <u>higher</u> than with preeclampsia.*

F. HELLP syndrome, a type of severe preeclampsia, is characterized by three conditions: Hemolysis, Elevated Liver enzymes, and Low Platelets.

Table 7–1
Hypertensive Disorders in Pregnancy

Diagnosis	Criteria
Mild preeclampsia (PIH)	*HTN* (BP ≥ 140/90 mm Hg) *Proteinuria* (1−2+ dipstick or > 300 mg/24 hr)
Severe preeclampsia (PIH)	*HTN* (BP ≥ 160/110 mm Hg) *Proteinuria* (3−4+ dipstick or > 5 g/24 hr) *Mild PIH with other signs/symptoms:* headache, epigastric pain, visual changes, DIC, ↑ liver enzymes, cyanosis, oliguria, pulmonary edema, IUGR
Eclampsia	Unexplained *tonic-clonic seizures* with mild or severe preeclampsia
Uncomplicated chronic HTN	*Preexisting HTN* or HTN diagnosed ≥ 20 weeks or persisting ≥ 6 weeks postpartum
Chronic HTN with superimposed PIH	*Chronic HTN with* ↑ *BP or* ↑ *proteinuria* in last half of pregnancy
Transient HTN	*Isolated HTN* without proteinuria in last half of pregnancy
HELLP syndrome	*HTN* in the presence of **H**emolysis, **E**levated **L**iver enzymes, **L**ow **P**latelets (HELLP)

BP = blood pressure
DIC = disseminated intravascular coagulation

HTN = hypertension
IUGR = intrauterine growth restriction

PIH = pregnancy-induced hypertension

III. RISK FACTORS: PREECLAMPSIA

A. **Demographic criteria: nulliparity (*most common* risk factor),** age extremes (< 20 years, > 34 years)

B. **Obstetric complications:** multiple gestation, molar pregnancy, nonimmune hydrops

C. **Medical complications:** diabetes mellitus (DM), chronic hypertension, preexisting renal disease, systemic lupus erythematosus

IV. PATHOGENESIS: PREECLAMPSIA

A. Diffuse vasospasm

1. Pathophysiology: increased production of thromboxane and decreased production of prostacyclin

2. Consequences: reduced perfusion of all organ systems, including the fetoplacental unit

B. Capillary wall injury, resulting in:

1. Vascular permeability, leading to hemoconcentration and edema

2. Disseminated intravascular coagulation (DIC), leading to fibrin deposition and platelet destruction

V. MANAGEMENT

A. Chronic hypertension

1. **Monitoring.** Outpatient conservative management is appropriate. Monthly ultrasonography will identify if IUGR develops. If IUGR is suspected, weekly NSTs or BPPs are indicated. Serial assessments of maternal BP and urine protein will identify superimposed preeclampsia.

2. **Medications.** With only mild to moderate hypertension and no end-organ damage, antihypertensive agents are not indicated since they do not improve perinatal outcomes. Antihypertensive therapy should be used for severe hypertension with methyldopa and labetalol as the first-line agents. Beta-blockers and diuretics may be used as secondary agents. ACE inhibitors are contraindicated during the second and third trimesters.

3. **Delivery.** Vaginal delivery at term is preferred for uncomplicated cases. Complicated or severe cases may be delivered early for maternal or fetal indications.

B. **Preeclampsia-eclampsia**

1. **Monitoring.** Initial in-hospital assessment of maternal and fetal condition is appropriate.
    a. **Mild preeclampsia** prior to 38 weeks' gestation can be managed on either an in-patient or outpatient (if reliable patient) basis with monitoring of maternal and fetal status.
    b. **Severe preeclampsia** and **eclampsia** are always managed in-hospital. Conservative management of severe preeclampsia between 23 and 32 weeks' gestation within an ICU setting with daily monitoring of mother and fetus may be appropriate in rare cases if no end-organ dysfunction or fetal jeopardy is present. All other cases are managed with immediate delivery.

2. **Medications**
    a. **Magnesium sulfate.** Seizure prophylaxis with IV $MgSO_4$ is used with mild preeclampsia only in labor. IV $MgSO_4$ (5 g loading dose over 20 minutes, then 2 g/hr maintenance) is used to stop seizures with eclampsia and prevent intrapartum seizures with all other preeclampsia patients.
    b. **Antihypertensive agents.** Hydralazine, labetalol, or nifedipine should be used to lower diastolic BP values between 90–100 mm Hg.
    c. **Corticosteroids.** For patients prior to 34 weeks' gestation, two doses of betamethasone (12 mg IM 24 hours apart) are administered to enhance fetal pulmonary surfactant.

3. **Delivery.** Vaginal delivery is preferred for all cases. Term delivery is appropriate for mild preeclampsia. Cesarean section delivery is used for only fetal and maternal indications.

C. **Preeclampsia superimposed on chronic hypertension** is managed with expeditious delivery due to the high rate of abruptio placenta and poor perinatal outcomes. Follow the guidelines for Medications and Delivery under Preeclampsia-Eclampsia above.

D. **Gestational hypertension**

1. **Monitoring.** Outpatient conservative management is appropriate. Appropriate fetal growth should be confirmed by ultrasound. If fetal status is determined reassuring with NST or BPP, no further fetal surveillance is needed. Frequent monitor of maternal BP and proteinuria is needed to identify developing preeclampsia.

2. **Medications.** No antihypertensive therapy is needed antepartum. $MgSO_4$ is not administered in labor.

3. **Delivery.** Vaginal delivery at term is appropriate. Cesarean section is performed only for maternal or fetal indications.

E. **HELLP syndrome** is managed with expeditious delivery due to the high rate of abruptio placentae and poor perinatal outcomes. Follow the guidelines for Medications and Delivery under Preeclampsia-Eclampsia above. Dexamethasone is administered to enhance normalization of abnormal laboratory parameters.

Clinical Situation 7–1

Basic Case: A 19-year-old primigravida at 32 weeks' gestation comes to the office for a routine prenatal visit. Her BP on a single measurement is 150/95 mm Hg. Her previous BPs have been 120/70–mm Hg range.

Patient Snapshot	Intervention	Clinical Pearls
She has lower extremity edema and swelling.	Repeat BP reading.	A diagnosis of HTN requires **sustained BP elevation.**
➤ After 15 minutes of left lateral rest: A second BP reading is 155/95 mm Hg.	Check urine protein.	**Gestational HTN** is diagnosed with sustained ↑ BP but no proteinuria.
➤ After 15 minutes of left lateral rest: A second BP reading is 155/95 mm Hg. Urine protein is 2+.	Must rule out pre-eclampsia.	**Mild preeclampsia** is diagnosed with HTN and $1-2+$ proteinuria.
➤ 1 hour later: ↑ BP persists, along with urine protein, 2+; Hgb, 13.0 g/dl; Hct, 38%; BUN, 12 mg/dl; creatinine, 1.1 mg/dl; uric acid, 8.0 mg/dl.	Admit and manage conservatively.	Prior to 36 weeks, mild preeclampsia is **managed conservatively.** Observe for progression to severe preeclampsia.
➤ At 34 weeks, after hospitalization for 2 weeks: BP is 160/110 mm Hg and 24-hr urine protein is 7.5 g. She has persistent headaches and epigastric pain.	Deliver promptly. Either vaginal delivery or CS may be appropriate.	**Severe preeclampsia** is managed by delivery regardless of gestational age. Lower diastolic BP to 90–100 mm Hg and start IV $MgSO_4$ for seizure prophylaxis.
➤ 1 hour later: induction of labor is begun, but before the IV $MgSO_4$ is given, she develops **tonic-clonic seizures.**	Administer IV $MgSO_4$ now.	**Eclampsia** is managed with IV $MgSO_4$ and prompt delivery regardless of gestational age.
➤ 2 hours later: while receiving IV $MgSO_4$ therapy, **her respirations have decreased from 20/min to 5/min.**	Stop $MgSO_4$. Give IV calcium gluconate.	These findings are consistent with **magnesium toxicity.** The antidote is IV calcium gluconate.

BP = blood pressure	Hgb = hemoglobin	HTN = hypertension
BUN = blood urea nitrogen	Hct = hematocrit	IV = intravenous
CS = cesarean section		

Clinical Situation 7–2

Basic Case: A 32-year-old multigravida comes to the office for a routine prenatal visit.

Patient Snapshot	Intervention	Clinical Pearls
At 16 weeks, her BP is 125/72 mm Hg but her urine dipstick shows 4+ proteinuria.	Order urinalysis and 24-hour urine protein collection.	**Chronic renal disease** is the most likely diagnosis with isolated proteinuria. Without ↑ BP, pre-eclampsia can be excluded.
At 16 weeks, her BP is 150/95 mm Hg with urine dipstick negative for protein.	Repeat BP after left lateral rest.	**Chronic HTN** is diagnosed with **sustained** ↑ BP < 20 weeks.
➡ 10 weeks later (26 weeks): With chronic HTN, BP is now 160/105 mm Hg. Urine protein is negative.	Start antihypertensive medication.	Diastolic BP ≥ 100 mm Hg should be treated. **Methyldopa** is the antihypertensive drug of choice.
➡ 14 weeks later (30 weeks) [on methyldopa]: BP is 155/95 mm Hg and urine protein is negative. NST is reactive and AFI is 10 cm.	Manage conservatively.	**Chronic HTN** prior to term is managed conservatively if the condition of the mother and fetus is reassuring.
➡ 3 weeks later (33 weeks): BP is sustained at 170/115 mm Hg, and 24-hr urine protein has increased from 1.2 to 8.3 g.	Deliver promptly.	**Chronic HTN with superimposed preeclampsia** is indication for delivery at any gestational age.
At 31 weeks, her BP is 140/90 mm Hg. Lab results are: Hgb, 7.0 g/dl; total bilirubin, 4.0 mg/dl; ALT, 400 U/dl; platelets, 85,000/µl.	Deliver promptly.	**HELLP syndrome** is indication for delivery at any gestational age.

AFI = amniotic fluid index	BP = blood pressure	HTN = hypertension
ALT = alanine aminotransferase	HELLP = hemolysis, elevated liver enzymes, low platelets	NST = nonstress test

8

Diabetes in Pregnancy

I. OVERVIEW

A. Significance. Diabetes mellitus (DM), which complicates 3% of all pregnancies, is characterized by glucose intolerance.

B. Classification

1. The **current division** into three groups is **based on pathophysiology (Table 8–1).**
   a. **Gestational diabetes mellitus (GDM)** is the *most common* of the three types. GDM results in insulin resistance from increasing levels of placental human placental lactogen (hPL) and insulinase. The overwhelming majority of cases are true pregnancy-induced GDM, but a minority are new-onset type 1 or type 2 DM that occurs during pregnancy.
   b. **Type 1 DM** results from **pancreatic islet cell destruction,** leading to **insulinopenia.**
   c. **Type 2 DM** results from **insulin resistance.**

2. The **White classification** system of several groups is based on disease duration and end-organ pathology.
   a. **Class A1:** gestational diabetes managed by diet alone
   b. **Class A2:** gestational diabetes requiring insulin
   c. **Class B:** diabetes onset < age 20 with duration < 10 years; no vascular complications
   d. **Class C:** diabetes onset age 10–19 years or duration 10–19 years; no vascular complications
   e. **Class D:** diabetes onset < age 10 years or duration > 20 years; vascular complications present
   f. **Class F:** presence of diabetic nephropathy
   g. **Class R:** presence of proliferative retinopathy
   h. **Class T:** presence of renal transplant
   i. **Class H:** presence of arteriosclerotic heart disease

II. COMPLICATIONS

A. Maternal complications. Individuals with type 1 DM uniquely are at risk for **ketoacidosis** and **hypoglycemic coma,** as opposed to patients with other types of DM. Other maternal complications may occur either before or during birth.

1. **Antepartum conditions**
   a. **Polyhydramnios** is *most common* in pregnant women with DM who have poor glycemic control.
   b. The risk of **preeclampsia** is increased.

Table 8–1

Types of Diabetes Mellitus in Pregnancy

	Gestational Diabetes Mellitus	Type 1 Diabetes Mellitus	Type 2 Diabetes Mellitus
Common name	Pregnancy-induced	Juvenile-onset	Adult-onset
Time of diagnosis	*Last half* of pregnancy	*Prior* to pregnancy	*Prior* to pregnancy
Mechanism	*Insulin resistance*	Insulin deficiency	*Insulin resistance*
Plasma insulin levels	High	Low	High
Risk of fetal anomalies	*Unchanged*	Increased	Increased

2. Intrapartum conditions
   a. Dysfunctional labor may be seen, with an overdistended uterus.
   b. Fetal macrosomia may lead to traumatic delivery, operative delivery, or cesarean section.

B. Fetal complications

   1. Congenital anomalies
      a. Anomalies are *most common* in women with **uncontrolled DM.** Risk is mediated through **hyperglycemia during embryogenesis** (weeks 2–8 postconception).
      b. Neural tube defects (NTDs) and **cardiac abnormalities** are the *most common* **anomalies. Sacral agenesis** (caudal regression syndrome) is the **most specific anomaly** for women with type 1 and type 2 DM.

   2. Growth disorders
      a. Macrosomia is the *most common* **growth disorder** seen in both GDM and preexisting DM.
      b. Intrauterine growth restriction (IUGR) may occur with maternal **small-vessel disease** (long-standing type 1 DM).

   3. Intrauterine compromise. Fetal jeopardy is mediated by the inability of the placenta to meet the requirements of a macrosomic fetus. The outcome may be **hypoxia** or even **fetal death.**

   4. Shoulder dystocia
      a. Impaction of the fetal anterior shoulder behind the maternal symphysis pubis is more common with macrosomia.
      b. Excessive lateral traction on the fetal head may result in **brachial plexus injury.**
      c. Management involves abduction/flexion of maternal thighs, suprapubic pressure, lateral rotation of the anterior shoulder, or delivery of the posterior arm.

C. Neonatal complications, which are largely caused by fetal hyperinsulinemia and immaturity

   1. Hypoglycemia due to persistent fetal **hyperinsulinemia** (from in utero hyperglycemia), which drives glucose downward

   2. Macrosomia due to fetal **hyperinsulinemia,** which increases fetal cellular intake of nutritional substrates

   3. Polycythemia due to relative intrauterine hypoxia, which causes increased erythropoietin

   4. Hyperbilirubinemia due to **immature** liver enzymes and breakdown of the increased red blood cells (RBCs) of polycythemia

5. Respiratory distress due to **immature** neonatal pulmonary surfactant production

6. Hypocalcemia due to **immature** parathyroid function

III. GOALS AND MODES OF THERAPY (same for both GDM and overt DM)

A. Target glucose values in the **euglycemic** range

   1. Fasting blood sugar (FBS) < 90 mg/dl

   2. 1-hour post-meal < 140 mg/dl

   3. 2-hour post-meal < 120 mg/dl

B. Dietary therapy

   1. Dietary goals for all diabetics are:

   a. Even distribution of calories over three meals per day and bedtime snack

   b. High-fiber foods and complex carbohydrates

   2. GDM can be managed by diet alone in 85% of cases.

C. Insulin management. Use subcutaneous human insulin for individuals with overt DM and for those with GDM who fail diet therapy. Total daily dose is calculated on actual body weight in kg.

   1. Starting dose: 0.8 U/kg (first trimester), 1.0 U/kg (second trimester), and 1.2 U/kg (third trimester)

   2. Split dose: two-thirds in the morning (two-thirds NPH and one-third regular insulin) and one-third in the evening (one-half NPH and one-half regular insulin)

   3. During labor: intravenous (IV) infusion (10 U regular insulin in 1 L D_5W), keeping glucose values between 80 and 100 mg/dl

   4. Postpartum insulin: discontinuation of the IV infusion after placental delivery to prevent hypoglycemia from rapid loss of the placental hormone effect. The prepregnancy insulin dose can be restarted in overt DM.

D. Oral hypoglycemic agents are **contraindicated** during pregnancy because of fetal nephrotoxicity.

IV. GESTATIONAL DIABETES MELLITUS (GDM)

A. Risk factors

   1. Positive family history

   2. Demographic factors: obesity, age > 25 years

   3. Maternal complications in previous pregnancy: unexplained stillbirth, traumatic delivery, shoulder dystocia

   4. Complications in previous infant: congenital anomaly, macrosomia, birth trauma

   5. Complications in current pregnancy: polyhydramnios, macrosomia, fetal anomaly

B. Screening involves the use of a **1-hour 50-gram oral glucose tolerance test (OGTT)** performed at 24–28 weeks.

   1. Normal glucose challenge result: **< 140 mg/dl**

   2. Necessity for a 3-hour 100-gram OGTT: ≥ 140 mg/dl

C. Diagnosis is based on an abnormal **3-hour 100-gram OGTT.** GDM is diagnosed if at least two of the following four values are elevated. Normal values are:

    1. FBS: < 95 mg/dl

    2. 1-hour: < 180 mg/dl

    3. 2-hour: < 155 mg/dl

    4. 3-hour: < 140 mg/dl

D. Management during pregnancy is based on the degree of glycemic control as well as maternal and fetal well-being.

    1. Initiate maternal dietary education and home blood glucose monitoring.

    2. Use conservative management with diet alone if glucose values are within the target range.

    3. Start insulin injections if glucose values are consistently above the target range.

    4. Monitor fetal growth and well-being with periodic fetal sonograms and biophysical profiles (BPPs).

    5. Begin twice-weekly nonstress tests (NSTs) and amniotic fluid indices (AFIs) at 32 weeks if a previous pregnancy ended in stillbirth, insulin is required, or the fetus is macrosomic.

    6. Watch for shoulder dystocia in labor. Consider cesarean delivery if estimated fetal weight (EFW) exceeds 4000–4500 g.

V. TYPES 1 AND 2 DIABETES MELLITUS (DM) [overt DM]

A. Screening for end-organ disease

    1. Kidney: 24-hour urine protein and creatinine clearance

    2. Retina: funduscopic examination after pupillary dilation

    3. Neuropathy: detailed neurologic examination

B. Fetal anomalies

    1. Risk of fetal anomalies (see II B 1–4)

    2. Detection of anomalies
        a. Sonogram at 10–12 weeks to identify anencephaly
        b. Triple marker screen at 15–20 weeks to screen for NTDs
        c. Sonogram at 18–20 weeks to screen for all anomalies
        d. Fetal echocardiogram at 22–24 weeks to screen for cardiac anomalies

    3. Prevention of anomalies
        a. Maintain **euglycemia** from preconception at least through the first trimester.
        b. Give folic acid supplementation (4 mg/day).

C. Management during pregnancy is based on the degree of glycemic control as well as maternal and fetal well-being.

    1. Initiate maternal dietary education and home blood glucose monitoring.

    2. Start subcutaneous human insulin injections.

    3. Monitor fetal growth and well-being with periodic fetal sonograms and BPPs.

    4. Begin twice-weekly NSTs and AFIs at 32 weeks (with no risk factors) or 26 weeks if vasculopathy, hypertension, or poor glucose control are present.

    5. Deliver no later than 40 weeks. Watch for shoulder dystocia in labor. Consider cesarean delivery if EFW exceeds 4000 g.

Clinical Situation 8–1

Basic Case: A 29-year-old multigravida is now 26 weeks' gestation by dates.

Patient Snapshot	Intervention	Clinical Pearls
A 1-hr 50-g Glucola screen is performed; the reported result is 155 mg/dl.	Perform a 3-hr 100-g OGTT.	Only 15% of gravidas with a **positive Glucola screen** (≥ 140 mg/dl) have a positive 3-hr 100-g OGTT.
➤ 4 days later: A 3-hr OGTT is performed; the reported results are: FBS, 89 mg/dl; **1-hr, 195 mg/dl; 2-hr, 165 mg/dl;** 3-hr, 135 mg/dl.	Initiate patient education concerning a diabetic diet and home glucose monitoring.	**GDM** is diagnosed when at least two of four values on the 3-hr OGTT are exceeded (FBS ≥ 95 mg/dl; 1-hr ≥ 180 mg/dl; 2-hr ≥ 155 mg/dl; and 3-hr ≥ 140 mg/dl).
➤ 2 weeks later (28 weeks): Her mean home glucose values are fasting, 85 mg/dl; and 1-hr post-meal, 130 mg/dl.	Observe because glucose values are in target range.	**Intervention is unnecessary** with GDM up to 40 weeks **if there are no risk factors** (diet therapy, normal fetal size, normal BP, no previous fetal demise).
➤ 2 weeks later (30 weeks): Her mean home glucose values are fasting, **105 mg/dl; 1-hr post-meal, 150 mg/dl.**	Start twice daily mixed dose (regular and NPH) insulin injections.	If **dietary therapy fails** to achieve target glucose values (FBS < 90 mg/dl, 1-hr post-meal < 140 mg/dl), **insulin therapy** is begun.
➤ 2 weeks later (32 weeks): She is still on insulin. Sonogram shows fetal growth at **95th percentile** of expected.	Start twice weekly NST and AFI fetal surveillance.	**Fetal surveillance** is started because the following risk factors are present: insulin therapy and macrosomia.
➤ 7 weeks later (39 weeks): She is still on insulin with sonographic EFW of 4600 g.	Plan primary cesarean delivery.	Avoid vaginal delivery because **shoulder dystocia** is markedly ↑ in diabetic pregnancies, with EFW > 4500 g.
➤ 1 day later: She undergoes an uncomplicated low-segment transverse primary cesarean delivery.	Give insulin on a sliding scale based on glucose values.	If the insulin dose is not markedly reduced postpartum, the rapid decrease in insulin resistance as hPL drops, possibly can cause **maternal hypoglycemia.**
➤ Her newborn son weighs 4500 g and has 1- and 5-minute Apgar scores of 8 and 9.	Monitor the infant closely.	**Infants of diabetic mothers** are at increased risk for ↓ glucose, ↓ calcium, ↑ bilirubin, ↑ Hct, and respiratory distress syndrome.
➤ 6 weeks after delivery: She returns for her check-up. She has not been on insulin since delivery. She is not breastfeeding.	Perform a 2-hr 75-g OGTT.	**Type 2 DM** is diagnosed if glucose intolerance persists, with FBS ≥ 126 mg/dl and other values ≥ 200 mg/dl.

AFI = amniotic fluid index   BP = blood pressure   DM = diabetes mellitus
EFW = estimated fetal weight   FBS = fasting blood sugar GDM = gestational diabetes mellitus
Hct = hematocrit   hPL = human placental lactogen   NST = nonstress test
OGTT = oral glucose tolerance test

9

Other Medical Complications in Pregnancy

I. ANEMIA

A. Definition. Anemia is a condition characterized by a **decrease in oxygen-carrying capacity.**

   1. Hemoglobin normal range in **nonpregnant state:** 13–15 g/dl

   2. Hemoglobin normal range in **pregnancy:** 10–12 g/dl, due to a greater expansion of plasma volume (50%) than red blood cell (RBC) mass (30%)

   3. Anemia in pregnancy: hemoglobin < 10 g/dl

B. Nutritional anemias. These disorders involve the **heme** part of the hemoglobin molecule.

   1. Iron-deficiency anemia is the *most common* anemia in women due to increased requirements from pregnancy and menstruation. No fetal impact is seen because active iron transport occurs across the placenta.

     a. Risk factors: frequent pregnancies, multiple gestation, poor nutrition, chronic bleeding

     b. Diagnosis: microcytic, hypochromic RBCs with a mean corpuscular volume (MCV) < 80 μm^3

     c. Prevention: elemental iron 30 mg/day

     d. Treatment: $FeSO_4$ 325 mg PO tid

   2. Folate-deficiency anemia is the second *most common* anemia.

     a. Risk factors: same as for iron-deficiency anemia (see I B 1 a), plus seizure medication, chronic hemolytic anemias

     b. Diagnosis: macrocytic RBC with MCV > 100 μm^3, hypersegmented neutrophils, decreased RBC folate

     c. Prevention: folic acid 0.4 mg/day PO

     d. Treatment: folic acid 1 mg/day

C. Inherited anemias. These disorders involve the **globin** part of the hemoglobin molecule.

   1. Sickle cell disease involves normal production of an **abnormal** hemoglobin chain (hemoglobin S).

     a. Risk factor. Sickle cell disease occurs almost exclusively in individuals of black African descent.

     b. Sickle cell trait. The **heterozygous state (SA)** has no fetal or neonatal effect. The only maternal impact is increased urinary tract infections (UTIs).

     c. Sickle cell anemia. The **homozygous state (SS)** results in significant anemia and RBC deformation with hypoxia. Treatment may require hospitalization and RBC transfusion. Hypoxia and iron overload should be avoided.

(1) Maternal complications: sickle cell crises, congestive heart failure, preeclampsia, infections, even death

(2) Perinatal complications: intrauterine growth restriction (IUGR), prematurity, stillbirth

2. **Thalassemia** involves impaired production of **normal α** or **β** hemoglobin chains. No treatment is available.

   a. **Risk factors.** Individuals of Southeast Asian, Mediterranean, or African descent are at risk for the disease.

   b. **α-Thalassemia minor.** Mild anemia is found in both the affected mother and fetus.

   c. **α-Thalassemia major. Hemoglobin Bart disease** causes severe fetal or neonatal anemia resulting in stillbirth or neonatal death.

   d. **β-Thalassemia minor.** Mild anemia is found in both the affected mother and fetus.

   e. **β-Thalassemia major. Cooley's anemia** causes severe childhood anemia resulting in either death or sterility.

II. CARDIAC DISEASE

A. Symptoms

1. **Severe dyspnea** (worsening dyspnea or paroxysmal nocturnal dyspnea)

2. **Orthopnea:** progressive

3. **Hemoptysis**

4. **Syncope** with exertion

5. **Chest pain** with effort or emotion

B. Signs

1. **Systolic murmur:** loud or pansystolic

2. **Diastolic murmur**

3. **Cardiomegaly,** including parasternal heave

4. **Cyanosis or clubbing**

5. **Jugular venous distention:** persistent

C. **New York Heart Association functional classification.** This system divides patients into four classes based on degree of maternal disability regardless of cardiac lesion.

1. **Low-risk patients** have a **good prognosis** and do not require invasive monitoring in labor.

   a. **Class I:** no cardiac decompensation

   b. **Class II:** no symptoms at rest, minor limitations with activity

2. **High-risk patients** have a **guarded prognosis** and require invasive monitoring in labor.

   a. **Class III:** no symptoms at rest, marked limitations with activity

   b. **Class IV:** symptoms even at rest

D. **Structural classification.** This system is based on the nature of the cardiac lesion.

1. **Acquired heart disease** (*most common* etiology is rheumatic)

   a. **Mitral stenosis** is the *most common* acquired heart disease in pregnancy. Complications arise from slowed diastolic filling across the stenotic valve, leading to left atrial enlargement, atrial fibrillation, and emboli.

   b. **Mitral insufficiency** is well-tolerated during pregnancy.

    2. Congenital heart disease

        a. **Atrial septal defect (ASD)** and **ventricular septal defect (VSD),** when taken together, are the *most common* **congenital heart lesions in adults.** They are usually tolerated well in pregnancy.

        b. **Tetralogy of Fallot** is the *most common* **cyanotic heart lesion in pregnancy.**

        c. **Marfan's syndrome** has a high maternal mortality rate if dilated aortic root ($>$ 40 mm).

        d. **Eisenmenger's syndrome** has a 50% maternal mortality rate. When systemic blood pressure drops, blood is shunted from the right to the left heart, bypassing the pulmonary circulation.

E. **Management of class III and IV heart disease in pregnancy.** Treatment seeks to offset the normal changes of pregnancy (increased blood volume, decreased heart rate) that increase stress on the heart.

    1. Antepartum measures

        a. **Limit intravascular fluid volume.** Encourage a low-sodium diet, and make free use of digitalis and diuretics.

        b. **Avoid tachycardia.** Restrict strenuous activity, and prevent anemia.

    2. Intrapartum measures

        a. **Monitor intravenous (IV) fluid volume.** Use an arterial line and pulmonary artery catheter.

        b. **Avoid tachycardia.** Provide reassurance, and use sedation and epidural anesthesia to control pain. Do not allow second-stage pushing.

        c. **Consider antibiotic prophylaxis** for subacute bacterial endocarditis (SBE).

            (1) **Use.** Antibiotics are **optional only** for vaginal delivery with previous SBE, a prosthetic heart valve, or complex congenital heart disease. They are **not recommended** for any cesarean delivery.

            (2) **Specific agents.** Ampicillin 2 g IV plus gentamicin 250 mg IV or vancomycin 1 g IV may be used.

    3. **Postpartum measures.** Watch for IV fluid volume **overload from** emptying of uterine venous sinuses, leading to **autotransfusion** of up to 400 ml of blood.

III. URINARY TRACT INFECTIONS (UTIs)

A. Overview

    1. UTIs are increased with pregnancy as a result of:

        a. Asymptomatic bacteriuria

        b. Physiologic urinary tract obstruction and stasis

        c. Pregnancy-induced glycosuria and amino acid aciduria

    2. Classification

        a. **Lower tract disease** involves only the bladder and urethra [e.g., asymptomatic bacteriuria (ASB), acute cystitis].

        b. **Upper tract disease** involves the kidneys (90% on the right side) [e.g., pyelonephritis].

B. **Pathophysiology. Pathogenic organisms ascending** from the vagina or rectum are the *most common* **source** of UTIs. *Escherichia coli* is the *most common* **causal organism** (70% of cases); other bacteria include *Klebsiella, Pseudomonas, Enterococcus,* and group B streptococcus.

C. Clinical entities

    1. **Asymptomatic bacteriuria (ASB)** is the *most common* **type of UTI** (8% incidence); the highest rates occur in pregnant women with the sickle cell trait. If ASB is untreated, 30% of cases progress to acute pyelonephritis.

   a. Diagnosis is **suspected** on the basis of pyuria and bacteriuria and is **confirmed** by a positive urine culture [> 100,000 CFU/ml of a single organism (not lactobacillus)].

   b. Treatment involves outpatient oral antibiotics (nitrofurantoin 100 mg PO bid for 7 days).

2. **Acute cystitis** is **symptomatic** (urgency, frequency, dysuria), but systemic physical findings are absent. **Diagnosis** and **treatment** are similar to ASB (see III C 1 a, b).

3. **Acute pyelonephritis** is the *most common* **serious medical complication** of pregnancy. In this systemic potentially life-threatening infection, bacteremia occurs in 15% of patients.

   a. Symptoms: chills, headache, flank pain, nausea, vomiting, preterm labor

   b. Diagnosis: fever, costovertebral angle (CVA) tenderness, dehydration, pyuria, bacteriuria, positive urine culture

   c. Treatment: hospitalization with parenteral antibiotics (cephalosporin 1–2 g IV q6hr) until temperature is normal and the CVA tenderness resolves

   (1) Oral outpatient treatment should be continued for 7 days.

   (2) Urine should be recultured after treatment to ensure eradication of the pathogen.

IV. OTHER MEDICAL COMPLICATIONS

A. Acute fatty liver of pregnancy. In this rare idiopathic condition, liver failure occurs with hypoglycemia and increased serum ammonia. This disorder can mimic severe preeclampsia with hypertension, proteinuria, edema, epigastric pain, and disseminated intravascular coagulation (DIC). Maternal mortality is 50%. **Treatment** involves supportive therapy in the intensive care unit.

B. Amniotic fluid embolism. In this rare condition, intravascular amniotic debris results in pulmonary hypertension, causing right-sided heart failure that leads to left-sided heart failure. It is almost always fatal. **Treatment** involves supportive therapy in the intensive care unit.

C. Cholestasis of pregnancy. Serum bile acids are elevated, causing severe itching. Because the risk for stillbirth and preterm delivery is increased with cholestasis, it is important to monitor fetal well-being with nonstress tests (NSTs) and amniotic fluid indices (AFIs) as well as to monitor for uterine contractions (UCs) and cervical dilation. **Treatment** is ursodeoxycholic acid with cholestyramine to lower bile acids and oral antihistamines for itching.

D. Deep venous thrombosis (DVT). Blood clots in pregnancy occur most commonly in the pelvic or lower extremity veins. The risk is markedly increased intrapartum and postpartum. DVT is diagnosed by duplex Doppler. **Treatment** is IV or subcutaneous heparin sufficient to double the partial thromboplastin time (PTT). Antepartum warfarin (Coumadin) should be avoided because of fetal risks.

E. Graves' disease. In this maternal autoimmune hyperthyroid condition, IgG antithyroid antibodies can also cross the placenta to the fetus. **Treatment** is propylthiouracil (PTU) or methimazole, using the lowest dose to restore euthyroidism because of possible adverse fetal effects.

F. Pruritic urticarial papules and plaques of pregnancy (PUPPP syndrome). This condition is the *most common* **pruritic dermatosis** of pregnancy. No adverse effect on pregnancy has been noted. Severe itching occurs along with a periumbilical rash that spreads to extremities. **Treatment** is with oral antihistamines and corticosteroids.

Clinical Situation 9–1

Basic Case: A 25-year-old multigravida comes to the office for a routine prenatal visit at 12 weeks' gestation. You review her prenatal laboratory panel.

Patient Snapshot	Intervention	Clinical Pearls
Her CBC shows an Hgb of **10.4 mg/dl.** Her RBC indices show an MCV of 92 μm^3 and an RDW of 12%.	Give iron 30 mg/day and folate 0.4 mg/day for **prophylaxis.**	Hemodilution of pregnancy results in an Hgb of 10–12 mg/dl. RBC indices are WNL.
Her CBC shows an Hgb of **9.1 mg/dl.** Her RBC indices show an MCV of 78 μm^3 and an RDW of 16%.	Give $FeSO_4$ 3 tablets per day as **treatment.**	With anemia and **microcytosis** the presumptive diagnosis is **iron deficiency,** the *most common* anemia in pregnancy.
Her CBC shows an Hgb of **9.1 mg/dl;** RBC indices show an MCV of 105 μm^3 and an RDW of 16%.	Give folic acid 1 mg per day as **treatment.**	With anemia and **macrocytosis,** the presumptive diagnosis is **folate-deficiency anemia.**
She is taking the appropriate treatment for her anemia. You want to assess whether her bone marrow is responding.	Order a reticulocyte count.	A rise in **reticulocyte count** occurs within 3 days, whereas a rise in hemoglobin may take 10–14 days.
She is of **southeast Asian descent.** She requests **thalassemia screening.**	Order hemoglobin electrophoresis.	**Electrophoresis** identifies homozygous or heterozygous deficiencies of either **alpha** or **beta hemoglobin** peptide chains.
She is of **African descent.** She requests **sickle cell screening.**	Order a sickle cell prep test.	This **screening test** only identifies whether hemoglobin S is present.
➔ The screening test is positive for **hemoglobin S.**	Order hemoglobin electrophoresis.	This **definitive test** differentiates between **homozygous** (> 40% Hgb S) and **heterozygous** (< 40% Hgb S) states.
➔ **Scenario 1** The Hgb electrophoresis identifies sickle cell trait (SA).	Screen for UTI.	The only perinatal complication with sickle cell trait is ↑ **asymptomatic bacteriuria** and ↑ cystitis.
➔ **Scenario 2** The Hgb electrophoresis identifies sickle cell anemia (SS).	Prevent hypoxia, folate deficiency, fetal jeopardy, and preterm labor.	Many maternal and fetal complications may occur. Perform serial sonograms for fetal growth, perform antepartum testing, and initiate preterm labor education.

CBC = complete blood count	RBC = red blood cell	UTI = urinary tract infection
Hgb = hemoglobin	RDW = red cell distribution width	WNL = within normal limits
MCV = mean corpuscular volume		

Clinical Situation 9–2

Basic Case: An 18-year-old primigravida at 36 weeks' gestation comes to the maternity unit in labor. She is having contractions every 3 minutes. The fetus is cephalic presentation, with the cervix 3 cm dilated, 90% effaced, and at −2 station.

Patient Snapshot	Intervention	Clinical Pearls
She has **unrepaired VSD.** Her prenatal course has been uncomplicated. She has worked throughout the pregnancy.	Give routine intrapartum care. No invasive monitoring is necessary.	**Class I heart disease** has no activity limitation. Women with ASD and VSD, even if unrepaired, do well in pregnancy.
She has **unrepaired tetralogy of Fallot.** Prenatally she had severe dyspnea and had to be hospitalized in the ICU. Now she complains of severe fatigue. Exam shows bilateral rales.	Induce labor with **invasive monitoring** in the cardiac ICU.	**Class III heart disease** results in symptoms with mild exertion. Uncorrected tetralogy of Fallot has a 10% maternal mortality rate. She needs prophylactic SBE antibiotics.
She has **Eisenmenger's syndrome.** She is having bright red vaginal bleeding and localized uterine tenderness. Her heart rate is 145 beats/min with a BP of 90/60 mm Hg.	Consider emergency cesarean section with **invasive monitoring.**	**The patient's mortality risk is 50%.** If her systemic pressure drops below her pulmonary pressure, and she shunts unoxygenated blood into her systemic circulation, she will die.

ASD = atrial septal defect   ICU = intensive care unit   VSD = ventricular septal defect
BP = blood pressure   SBE = subacute bacterial endocarditis

Clinical Situation 9–3

Basic Case: A 25-year-old multigravida at 25 weeks' gestation comes to the office for a routine prenatal visit.

Patient Snapshot	Intervention	Clinical Pearls
She has no symptoms of urgency or frequency. A urine culture shows *Escherichia coli* > 100,000 CFU/ml.	Give single-agent **outpatient** oral antibiotics.	**Asymptomatic bacteriuria** occurs in 8% of gravidas. If untreated, it progresses to pyelonephritis in 30% of cases.
She complains of urgency and frequency. She is afebrile. Physical exam is normal. A urine culture shows *E. coli* > 100,000 CFU/ml.	Give single-agent **outpatient** oral antibiotics.	**Acute cystitis** occurs in 1% of gravidas. If untreated, it progresses to pyelonephritis in 30% of cases.
She complains of right flank pain. She has a fever of 103°F. Physical exam confirms right CVA tenderness. Urinalysis shows clumps of WBCs and many bacteria.	**Hospitalize** with IV hydration and IV antibiotics.	**Pyelonephritis** is a life-threatening infection that must be treated aggressively. Watch for preterm labor. Discharge with prophylactic antibiotics to prevent recurrence.

CVA = costovertebral angle   IV = intravenous   WBC = white blood cell

10

Labor and Delivery

I. NORMAL LABOR

A. **Terminology used to describe in utero fetal orientation (Figure 10–1)**

1. **Lie** refers to the relationship between the long axis of the fetus and the long axis of the mother. The *most common* **lie** is **longitudinal;** the spine of the fetus is parallel to the spine of the mother.

2. **Presentation** refers to the fetal part that overlies the pelvic inlet. The *most common* **presentation** is **cephalic;** the fetal head overlies the pelvic inlet.

3. **Position** refers to the relationship between a reference point on the fetal presenting part and the maternal bony pelvis. The *most common* **position** is **occiput anterior;** the fetal posterior fontanelle lies in the anterior birth canal.

4. **Attitude** refers to the degree of extension or flexion of the fetal head. The *most common* **attitude** is **vertex;** the fetal head is flexed, with the chin against the chest.

5. **Station** refers to the degree of descent of the presenting part through the birth canal. Station is expressed as **minus** values (i.e., **above** the level of the ischial spines) or **plus** values (i.e., **below** the level of the ischial spines).

B. **Cardinal movements of labor.** These sequential changes in position and attitude of the fetal head, which are also known as the **mechanisms of labor,** occur during passage through the birth canal **(Table 10–1).** Although the first three movements are described separately, they occur virtually simultaneously.

C. **Stages of labor (Chart 10–1).** The onset of regular contractions to expulsion of the placenta is a sequential process that can be described in three stages **(Table 10–2).** The first stage is divided into latent and active phases.

D. **Obstetric analgesia.** Various modalities help the patient cope with the pain of labor. Each method has certain limitations and side effects **(Table 10–3).**

II. ABNORMAL LABOR. This can be classified into five types—either **prolongation** or **arrest** disorders **(Figure 10–2).**

A. Prolonged latent phase

1. **Definition:** duration > 14 hours in a multipara or > 20 hours in a primipara

2. **Etiology:** injudicious **analgesia; hypotonic uterine contractions (UCs)** [low intensity, short duration]; **hypertonic UCs** (high intensity, short duration)

3. **Management:** ambulation or sedation; avoidance of cesarean section or oxytocin

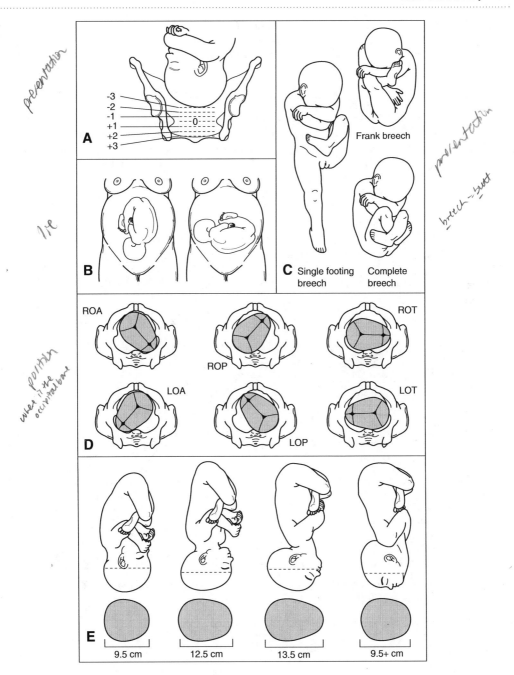

Figure 10–1. (*A*) Stations of the fetal head. (*B*) Longitudinal and transverse lies. (*C*) Types of breech presentation. (*D*) Various positions of the fetal head in a vertex presentation. (*E*) Types of cephalic presentation according to attitude of fetal head. (After Beckman CR, Ling FW, Barzansky BM et al: *Obstetrics and Gynecology*, 2nd ed. Baltimore, Williams & Wilkins, 1995, p 172; DeCherney AH, Pernoll ML [eds]: *Current Obstetrics & Gynecologic Diagnosis & Treatment*, 8th ed. East Norwalk, CT, Appleton & Lange, 1994, pp 214; and Scott JR, DiSaia PJ, Hammond CB et al [eds]: *Danforth's Obstetrics and Gynecology*, 6th ed. Philadelphia, JB Lippincott, 1990, pp 168, 170.)

Table 10–1
Cardinal Movements of Labor

Movement	Definition	Purpose
1. Engagement	Descent of fetal head (in transverse position) to below pelvic inlet plane	Demonstrates adequacy of pelvic inlet
2. Descent	Downward movement of fetus through curve of birth canal	Transports fetus from uterine cavity out of mother's body
3. Flexion	Movement of fetal chin toward thorax	Allows narrowest fetal head diameter to present to birth canal
4. Internal rotation	Rotation of fetal head within birth canal from transverse to AP	Allows widest fetal head diameter to present to widest part of the maternal bony pelvis
5. Extension	Movement of fetal chin away from thorax	Directs fetal head upward to pelvic outlet and out of mother's body
6. External rotation	Rotation of fetal head outside mother's body from AP to transverse	Allows fetal shoulders to present to widest diameter of mid pelvis
7. Expulsion	Emerging of remainder of fetus from mother's body	Completes birth process

AP = anterior-posterior

B. Prolonged active phase

1. Definition: inadequate change in cervical dilation (< 1.5 cm/hr in a multipara or < 1.2 cm/hr in a primipara)

2. Etiology (the "three Ps"): Pelvis (inadequate bony pelvis size); **Passenger** (excessive fetal size or abnormal fetal lie, presentation, position); **Powers** (inadequate UCs)

3. Management: intravenous (IV) oxytocin if UCs are inadequate (**duration:** < 45 seconds; **frequency:** < 3 in 10 minutes; **intensity:** < 50 mm Hg)

C. Active phase arrest

1. Definition: no change in cervical dilation for ≥ 2 hours

2. Etiology: problems with **Pelvis, Passenger, or Powers**

3. Management: IV oxytocin if UCs are inadequate; cesarean section if UCs are adequate or the mother fails to respond to oxytocin

D. Prolonged second stage (arrest of descent)

1. Definition: no delivery of fetus in spite of ≥ 2 hours of effective maternal pushing efforts

2. Etiology: problems with **Pelvis, Passenger, or Powers**

3. Management: IV oxytocin if UCs are inadequate; vacuum extraction, forceps-assisted delivery, or cesarean section if UCs are adequate or the UCs fail to respond to oxytocin

E. Prolonged third stage

1. Definition: placenta remains undelivered for 30 minutes after delivery of the fetus

Labor Stage	Definition	Duration
Stage 1 Latent Phase ***Effacement***	Begins: Onset of reg UC Ends: Accel of cerv dil *Prepares cervix for dilation*	< 20 hr in primipara < 14 hr in multipara
Stage 1 Active Phase ***Dilation***	Begins: Accel of cervical dilation Ends: 10 cm (complete) *Rapid Cervical Dilation*	≤ 1.2 cm/hr primip ≤ 1.5 cm/hr multip
Stage 2 ***Descent***	Begins: 10 cm (complete) Ends: Delivery of baby *Descent of fetus*	< 2 hr in primipara < 1 hr in multipara *Add 1 hr if epidural*
Stage 3 ***Expulsion***	Begins: Delivery of baby Ends: Delivery of placenta *Delivery of placenta*	< 30 minutes

UC = uterine contraction

Chart 10–1.

    2. Etiology: inadequate UCs; abnormal trophoblastic invasion (placenta accreta, increta, or percreta)

    3. Management: IV oxytocin if UCs are inadequate; manual placental removal

  F. Questions to ask in labor management

    1. Is the patient actually in labor? Look for progressive changes in cervical dilation.

    2. What stage of labor is the patient in (see Table 10–2)?

    3. Is the labor abnormal in any way? If so, determine the type of labor abnormality exhibited by the patient (see II A—E).

    4. Is the quality of UCs adequate (see II B 3)?

III. OPERATIVE DELIVERY. Certain obstetric procedures that involve active measures, (including forceps-assisted delivery, vacuum extractor delivery, and cesarean delivery), may be necessary to accomplish delivery.

Table 10–2
Stages of Labor

	Description	Purpose
Stage 1: latent phase	*Begins* with onset of regular UCs *Ends* at 3–4-cm dilation (acceleration of cervical dilation slope)	Coordination of UCs and cervical softening and effacement
Stage 1: active phase	*Begins* at 3–4-cm dilation *Ends* at 10-cm dilation (complete dilation)	Active cervical dilation, beginning of descent of fetus, and beginning of cardinal movements of labor
Stage 2	*Begins* at 10-cm dilation *Ends* with delivery of fetus	Completion of descent of fetus and completion of cardinal movements of labor
Stage 3	*Begins* with delivery of fetus *Ends* with delivery of placenta	Complete expulsion of all products of conception

UC = uterine contraction

A. Forceps delivery

    1. **Classification** of forceps is made according to fetal head position and station.

        a. **Outlet forceps.** The fetal head is on the pelvic floor and rotation is ≤ 45 degrees. Fetal and maternal risk is minimal.

        b. **Low forceps.** The fetal head is below +2 station but not on the pelvic floor. Fetal and maternal risk is minimal.

        c. **Mid forceps.** The fetal head is engaged (below 0 station) but has not reached +2 station. Fetal and maternal risk is greater.

        d. **High forceps.** The fetal head is unengaged (above 0 station). Fetal and maternal risk is so great that high forceps have no place in modern obstetrics.

Table 10–3
Obstetric Pain Relief

Modality	Description	Limitations
Natural method (Stage 1)	Focused concentration and controlled breathing	Much individual variability of pain relief
Narcotic use (Stage 1)	IM or IV injection of narcotics	*Neonatal respiratory depression* if delivery occurs within 30–60 minutes
Paracervical block (Stage 1)	Injection of anesthetic in vaginal fornices	*Fetal bradycardia* from high local anesthetic concentrations in utero
Epidural block (Stages 1 or 2)	Infusion of anesthetic into epidural space	*Maternal hypotension* from sympathetic blockade *Spinal headache* if dura is pierced
Local anesthesia (Stage 2)	Local anesthetic infiltration for suture repair	Inadequate relief if extensive repair necessary
Pudendal block (Stage 2)	Local anesthetic block of pudendal nerve near the ischial spine	Variable degree of pain relief

IM = intramuscular   IV = intravenous

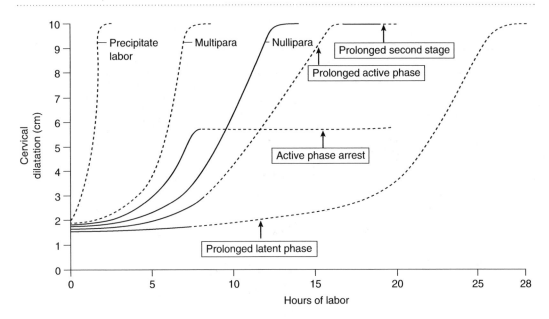

Figure 10–2.   Abnormal labor curves. (From DeCherney AH, Pernoll ML [eds]: *Current Obstetric & Gynecologic Diagnosis & Treatment*, 8th ed. East Norwalk, CT, Appleton & Lange, 1994, p 218.)

      2. Prerequisites include complete cervical dilation, ruptured membranes, engagement of the fetal head, and known orientation of the fetal head.

B. Cesarean delivery

    1. Indications: **primary cesarean**
       a. *Most common:* cephalopelvic disproportion (CPD), a generic term that denotes failure to follow a normal labor dilation curve (see Figure 10–2)
       b. Second most common: breech presentation

    2. Uterine incisions (Figure 10–3)
       a. The **low segment transverse incision** is the *most common* incision used because in subsequent pregnancy, labor is usually safe. In addition, the risk of blood loss and adhesion is less.
       b. The **classical incision** is not limited by fetal size or orientation, but in subsequent pregnancy, it has a 5% risk of rupture in labor. In addition, the risk of blood loss and adhesion is greater with the classical incision. It is used only rarely.
       c. The **low segment vertical incision** is seldom used. This incision may extend into upper segment.

C. Vaginal birth after previous cesarean (VBAC)

    1. VBAC is successful in up to 85% of patients in whom it is performed, depending on the indication for the primary cesarean delivery.

    2. A **previous low segment** uterine incision is the most important prerequisite. An incision in the uterine fundus (classical or extended low vertical) has a significant risk of catastrophic rupture and is a contraindication for labor.

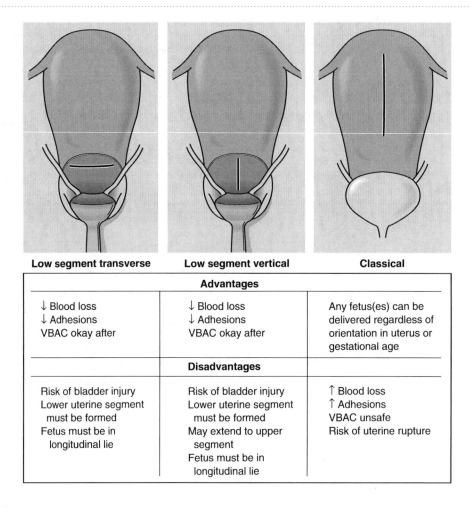

	Low segment transverse	Low segment vertical	Classical
Advantages	↓ Blood loss ↓ Adhesions VBAC okay after	↓ Blood loss ↓ Adhesions VBAC okay after	Any fetus(es) can be delivered regardless of orientation in uterus or gestational age
Disadvantages	Risk of bladder injury Lower uterine segment must be formed Fetus must be in longitudinal lie	Risk of bladder injury Lower uterine segment must be formed May extend to upper segment Fetus must be in longitudinal lie	↑ Blood loss ↑ Adhesions VBAC unsafe Risk of uterine rupture

Figure 10–3.   Comparison of uterine cesarean incisions. VBAC = vaginal birth after cesarean. (After Gabbe SG, Niebyl JR, Simpson JL [eds]: *Obstetrics: Normal and Problem Pregnancies*, 2nd ed. New York, Churchill Livingstone, 1991, p 646.)

   D. Vacuum extractor delivery

      1. A soft Silastic cup, held against the fetal head with a vacuum, is used to apply traction on the fetal head simultaneously with maternal second-stage pushing efforts.

      2. Indications and prerequisites are similar to those of forceps delivery (see III A 2), except that a **knowledge of the orientation of the position of the fetal head is less essential.**

Clinical Situation 10–1

Basic Case: A 32-year-old multigravida at 38 weeks' gestation in the maternity unit is under observation. She is having UCs every 3–5 minutes and appears uncomfortable.

Patient Snapshot	Intervention	Clinical Pearls
Her cervix is dilated 1–2 cm, 50% effaced, −2 station. This has remained essentially unchanged for the past 6 hours.	Consider ambulation or sedation. Avoid CS and oxytocin.	This is normal **latent phase** (cervical dilation < 3 cm), during which UCs coordinate and cervical effacement progresses.
➡ 6 hours later: She is in active labor at 4-cm dilation and has just received a paracervical block. The baseline FHR is now 90 beats/min.	Use conservative management.	**High local anesthetic concentrations** immediately after the paracervical block rapidly dilute, reversing the effect on the FHR.
➡ 2 hours later: Now she is 7 cm dilated, 80% effaced, −1 station. The EFM tracing is reassuring.	Observe.	The normal active phase **cervical dilation rate** for a multipara is 1.5 cm/hr and 1.2 cm/hr for a primipara.
➡ 1 hour later: She has just received an epidural anesthesia. Five minutes later, the FHR drops to 85 beats/min.	Administer a rapid IV bolus of isotonic fluids and IV ephedrine.	**Rapid sympathetic blockade** can result in vasodilation, hypotension, and placental hypoperfusion.
➡ 2 hours later: She has now been 7 cm dilated for the past 3 hours with no further change. The EFM tracing is reassuring	Assess quality of UCs.	If **active phase arrest** is caused by inadequate contractions, treatment is IV oxytocin augmentation.
➡ 5 hours later: After administration of IV oxytocin, she quickly progresses to 10-cm dilation. She has now been pushing for 3 hours, but the fetal head is still at +3 station.	Consider forceps, vacuum extractor, or CS.	With **second-stage arrest,** an operative vaginal delivery or an emergency CS may be indicated.
➡ She has just undergone a forceps-assisted vaginal delivery of a 3100-g male neonate with depressed respirations. She received IV meperidine 30 minutes ago.	Give the infant naloxone.	**Neonatal respiratory depression** is common if birth occurs shortly after maternal narcotics. Naloxone reverses the effect of narcotics.
➡ After delivery, she complains of an intense throbbing headache whenever she raises her head. It disappears if she lowers her head.	Give oral and IV hydration; caffeine; blood patch.	**Spinal headache** results from inadvertent dural puncture with the epidural. Sealing off the CSF fluid leakage stops the headache.

CS = cesarean section   EFM = electronic fetal monitoring   IV = intravenous
CSF = cerebrospinal fluid   FHR = fetal heart rate   UC = uterine contraction

Clinical Situation 10–2

Basic Case: A 25-year-old multigravida in stage 2 of labor is exhausted after pushing for 3 hours. The woman is 5' 6" tall and weighs 175 lb. The presentation is cephalic with an estimated fetal weight of 3500 g.

Patient Snapshot	Intervention	Clinical Pearls
The fetal head position is **occiput anterior with station at +3** on the pelvic floor. Pelvic capacity appears adequate.	Use outlet forceps or vacuum extractor.	**Outlet forceps delivery:** the fetal head is on the pelvic floor and rotation is ≤ 45°. Fetal and maternal risk is minimal.
The fetal head position is **left occiput transverse with station at +1.**	Use trial of mid-forceps or CS if forceps fail.	**Mid-forceps delivery:** the fetal head is engaged (below 0 station) but not down to the pelvic floor. Fetal and maternal risk is greater.
The fetal head position is **right occiput posterior with station at −2.**	Perform emergency CS (no trial of forceps!).	**High forceps delivery:** the fetal head is unengaged (above 0 station). Fetal and maternal risk is so great that high forceps have no place in modern obstetrics.

CS = cesarean section

Clinical Situation 10–3

Basic Case: A 29-year-old multigravida comes to the office for a routine prenatal visit. Fetal heart tones are within normal limits, and fundal height is appropriate for gestational age. She has no uterine contractions, and on pelvic exam, her cervix is closed.

Patient Snapshot	Intervention	Clinical Pearls
Gestational age is **27 weeks.** Fetal presentation is **complete breech.**	Use conservative management.	A breech fetus is a normal event at this gestational age. Spontaneous version will probably occur.
Gestation age is **37 weeks.** Fetal presentation is **complete breech.**	Consider external version; discuss CS.	Spontaneous version from breech is common before 37 weeks. Amniotic fluid decreases after 37 weeks.
Gestational age is **37 weeks.** Fetal presentation is **frank breech.**	Consider vaginal delivery, external version, or discuss CS.	For safe vaginal breech delivery, ensure pelvic adequacy by CT pelvimetry. Also, the fetal head must not be extended.

CS = cesarean delivery   CT = computed tomography

Clinical Situation 10–4

Basic Case: A 28-year-old multigravida at 37 weeks' gestation comes to the maternity unit with regular uterine contractions. Her cervix is 3 cm dilated.

Patient Snapshot	Intervention	Clinical Pearls
Fetal presentation is **frank breech.** Both thighs are flexed, but the legs are extended.	Perform emergency CS or vaginal delivery.	A frank breech is the **only breech presentation** that may be **safe for vaginal delivery.** A CS is also a reasonable choice.
Fetal presentation is **complete breech.** Both thighs are flexed and the knees are bent.	Perform emergency CS (unsafe for vaginal delivery).	Complete breech is **unstable,** because extension of the fetal knees leads to a footling breech.
Fetal presentation is **footling breech.** Both thighs and knees are extended.	Perform emergency CS (unsafe for vaginal delivery).	Footling breech is dangerous because although the feet and body deliver without problems, the **after-coming head could become trapped.**

CS = cesarean section

Clinical Situation 10–5

Basic Case: A 34-year-old multigravida who delivered her previous baby by CS now comes to the maternity unit at 38 weeks' gestation with regular UCs. Her cervix is 3 cm dilated.

Patient Snapshot	Intervention	Clinical Pearls
The previous CS involved a **classical uterine incision.**	Perform emergency repeat CS.	Classical uterine incisions have a significant chance of **catastrophic rupture.** Labor and vaginal delivery are unsafe.
The previous CS involved a **low vertical uterine incision.**	Perform emergency repeat CS or VBAC.	Repeat CS and VBAC are both safe options if the vertical incision **did not extend into the fundus.**
The previous CS involved a **low transverse uterine incision.**	Perform emergency repeat CS or VBAC.	With a low transverse uterine incision, repeat **CS and vaginal delivery are both safe options.** The choice is up to the patient.

UC = uterine contraction   CS = cesarean section   VBAC = vaginal birth after cesarean

11

Labor and Delivery Complications

I. PREMATURE RUPTURE OF MEMBRANES (PROM)

A. Overview

    1. Definitions

      a. **PROM:** rupture of the amnion and chorion prior to the onset of labor

      b. **Preterm PROM (PPROM):** rupture of the amnion and chorion prior to 36 weeks

    2. **Significance.** PROM is the single *most common* **diagnosis** leading to neonatal intensive care unit admissions.

B. **Diagnostic criteria on speculum examination** (all must be present)

    1. **Pooling of amniotic fluid** in the posterior vaginal fornix

    2. **Nitrazine paper** that turns blue when placed in alkaline amniotic fluid taken from the fornix. (Bloody fluid can give false-positive results.)

    3. **Ferning pattern** seen with microscope when amniotic fluid from the posterior fornix dries on a glass slide

C. **Risk factors**

    1. **Ascending infection** from lower genital tract

    2. **Serial damage** to membranes from uterine contractions (UCs)

    3. **Local defects** within the membranes

    4. **Cigarette smoking**

D. Hazards associated with PROM (Chart 11–1)

    1. Complications if the fetus remains in the uterus

      a. **Neonatal conditions:** infection and sepsis, deformations, umbilical cord compression, pulmonary hypoplasia

      b. **Maternal conditions:** chorioamnionitis, sepsis, deep venous thrombosis (DVT), psychosocial separation from family

    2. Complications if premature delivery occurs. The following **neonatal conditions** are inversely related to gestational age:

      a. **Respiratory distress syndrome (RDS):** *most common* **morbidity** in premature infants

      b. Patent ductus arteriosus (PDA)

      c. Intraventricular hemorrhage (IVH)

      d. Necrotizing enterocolitis (NEC)

      e. Retinopathy of prematurity (ROP)

Hazards associated with PROM

If fetus remains in utero	If preterm delivery occurs
Neonatal conditions • infection & sepsis • deformations • umbilical cord compress • pulmonary hypoplasia	**Neonatal conditions** • **RDS** (most common) • **PDA** (patent ductus arteriosus) • **IVH** (intraventricular hemorrhage) • **NEC** (necrotizing enterocolitis) • **ROP** (retinopathy of prematurity) • **BPD** (bronchopulmonary dysplasia) • **CP** (cerebral palsy)
Maternal conditions • chorioamnionitis, sepsis • deep venous thrombosis (DVT) • psychosocial separation	

PROM = premature rupture of fetal membrane

Chart 11–1.

       f. Bronchopulmonary dysplasia
       g. Cerebral palsy

E. Management
   1. Complicated PROM. Prompt delivery should occur in the presence of the following conditions:
     a. Fetal lung maturity: lecithin/sphingomyelin (L/S) ratio > 2 on analysis of pooled vaginal amniotic fluid or TDX-FLM test is mature.
     b. Chorioamnionitis: maternal fever unexplained by an upper respiratory infection (URI) or urinary tract infection (UTI) [start therapeutic antibiotics (clindamycin 900 mg IV q8hr and gentamicin 250 mg IV q24hr)]
     c. Fetal jeopardy: nonreassuring electronic fetal monitoring (EFM) strip or biophysical profile (BPP) [emergency cesarean section may be necessary]
   2. Uncomplicated PROM. Treatment varies according to **gestational age.**
     a. Term (≥ 36 weeks). The **goal is delivery,** because prolonging the pregnancy has no maternal or fetal benefit. Depending on clinical presentation, labor should be induced with oxytocin or a cesarean section should be performed.
     b. Preterm (24–35 weeks). The **goal is prolongation of pregnancy** to minimize the many neonatal risks of prematurity. The patient should be transferred to a perinatal center for in-hospital conservative management. The following measures may be effective.
     (1) Bed rest: leg exercises to prevent thrombosis
     (2) Prophylactic antibiotics [used after obtaining vaginal/cervical cultures, specifically looking for group B β-hemolytic Streptococcus (GBBS)]: ampicillin (2 g IV q6hr) and erythromycin (250 mg IV q6hr) for 48 hours, then both orally for 5 days

(3) **Maternal corticosteroids** to accelerate fetal lung maturity prior to 32 weeks: two doses of betamethasone (12 mg IM) 24 hours apart

(4) **Monitoring of fetal well-being:** serial nonstress tests (NSTs) and BPPs

c. **Previable** (< 24 weeks). The **goal is maternal safety,** because the likelihood of perinatal survival is low. The patient should be offered the following options:

(1) **Induction of labor:** intravenous (IV) oxytocin

(2) **Home management:** bed rest

II. PRETERM LABOR AND DELIVERY

A. Incidence

1. Approximately 10% of all deliveries occur prior to 37 completed weeks of gestation.

2. Preterm delivery is the **most common** cause of neonatal deaths in the United States. In spite of extensive use of tocolytic agents, no reduction in preterm delivery rates has occurred in the past 50 years. Most patients receiving tocolytics are not in preterm labor but are having preterm contractions.

B. **Risk factors** for preterm delivery

1. **Lifestyle:** smoking, heavy physical labor

2. **Obstetric history: previous preterm birth,** previous second-trimester abortion

3. **Current pregnancy: uterine anomaly, multiple gestation,** short cervix, bacterial vaginosis, trichomonas vaginitis, periodontal gum disease

C. **Criteria for diagnosis of preterm labor** (all must be present)

1. **Gestational age:** between 20 and 37 weeks

2. **Contractions:** ≥ 3 UCs (lasting ≥ 30 seconds) in 20 minutes

3. **Cervical dilation:** ≥ 2 cm (single examination) or a change in dilation/effacement (serial examinations)

D. **Criteria for diagnosis of preterm contractions**

1. **Gestational age** and **frequency of contractions** [same as in preterm labor (see II C 1, 2)]

2. **No change in cervical dilation/effacement** on serial examination

E. **Contraindications for tocolysis.** In certain circumstances, attempts to prolong the pregnancy are either futile or hazardous to the fetus or the mother.

1. **Fetal conditions:** fetal demise, fetal distress, severe intrauterine growth restriction (IUGR), lethal anomaly

2. **Maternal conditions:** severe preeclampsia, eclampsia, uncontrolled diabetes mellitus (DM), advanced cervical dilation

3. **Placental/membrane-related conditions:** spontaneous rupture of membranes (SROM), severe abruptio placentae, unstable placenta previa, chorioamnionitis

F. **Tocolytic agents.** These substances can be expected to delay delivery for only 24–48 hours.

1. Magnesium sulfate
   a. **Mechanism:** competes for Ca^{2+} during muscle depolarization
   b. **Side effects:** pulmonary edema, muscle weakness, respiratory depression
   c. **Dose:** loading dose of 5 g IV, then 1–4 g/hr as needed

  2. **β-adrenergic agonists (ritodrine, terbutaline)**
      a. **Mechanism:** stimulates β receptors to relax smooth muscle
      b. **Side effects:** pulmonary edema, hypotension, tachycardia, hyperglycemia, hypokalemia (intracellular K$^+$ shift)
      c. **Dose**
          (1) Ritodrine: 100 μg/min IV to start, increasing to 350 μg/min as needed
          (2) Terbutaline: 0.25 mg SQ q1–4hr as needed

  3. **Prostaglandin synthetase inhibitors (indomethacin)** [seldom used because of serious fetal side effects]
      a. **Mechanism:** inhibits prostaglandin synthesis and release
      b. **Side effects:** fetal PDA closure (highest risk after 32 weeks), oligohydramnios, increased neonatal NEC
      c. **Dose:** 50–100 mg rectal suppository; then 25 mg PO q6hr for 24 hours

  4. **Calcium channel blockers (nifedipine)**
      a. **Mechanism:** causes decrease in intracellular Ca^{2+} ions
      b. **Side effects:** hypotension, tachycardia, myocardial depression
      c. **Dose:** starting dose of 5 mg PO up to 40 mg as needed, then 10–20 mg q4hr

G. Management of preterm labor

  1. **Confirm presence** of all criteria for **preterm labor.**

  2. **Confirm** maternal and fetal **well-being.**

  3. **Confirm absence** of contraindications to tocolysis.

  4. **Obtain** vaginal and urine culture for GBBS and start IV pen G.

  5. **Initiate tocolysis** using the lowest dose to achieve suppression of contractions.
      a. **Administer maternal betamethasone** prior to 34 weeks to accelerate fetal lung maturity.
      b. **Transfer the patient** to a perinatal center with a neonatal intensive care nursery.

III. POSTDATES PREGNANCY

A. Overview

  1. **Definition** (assuming a 28-day menstrual cycle): a pregnancy persisting postconception for 40 weeks (280 days) or post–last menstrual period (LMP) for 42 weeks (294 days)

  2. **Confounding factors**
      a. The menstrual cycles of most women are not 28 days in length.
      b. Frequently, the date of conception or even the LMP is uncertain.

B. **Perinatal hazards.** The effect of pregnancy prolongation on placental functioning may lead to problems. Two possible scenarios may occur.

  1. **Macrosomia syndrome,** the *most common* outcome (75% of cases), occurs if **placental function is maintained.** Complications of a large uterus include arrest of labor and cesarean delivery or traumatic vaginal delivery.

  2. **Dysmaturity syndrome** (25% of cases) may be seen if **placental aging** develops. This condition leads to placental insufficiency (decreased nutritional supply, reduced oxygenation). Complications include fetal hypoxia and meconium aspiration syndrome.

C. **Accuracy of pregnancy dating.** Accurate determination is critical. Review of prenatal records identifies the following factors that provide confidence in gestational age.

1. **Accurate menstrual history:** certain LMP, planned pregnancy, normal menstrual cycle

2. **Documentation of early pregnancy landmarks:** early fetal heart tones (FHTs) by Doppler or fetuscope or early fetal movements

3. **Early sonogram:** accurate ± 5 days at less than 12 weeks, ± 7 days from 12–18 weeks

D. **Management of suspected postdates pregnancy**

1. Determine your confidence in the gestational age dating.

2. Establish how favorable the cervix is (dilated, effaced, soft).

3. Assess fetal well-being [e.g., with NSTs and amniotic fluid indices (AFIs)]. If fetal jeopardy is evident, immediate delivery is appropriate.

4. Use the following triage method.
   a. **Dates are certain and the cervix is favorable.** Neither the mother nor the fetus benefits from waiting. **Induce labor promptly** with IV oxytocin and rupture of membranes.
   b. **Dates are certain but the cervix is unfavorable.** The risk of failed induction is high. If fetal macrosomia is suspected, **induce labor** with prostaglandin PGE_2. Alternatively, if the estimated fetal weight (EFW) is normal, **manage expectantly** with twice-weekly NSTs and AFIs.
   c. **Dates are unsure.** Because it is not known if the patient is postdates, delivery is not indicated. **Manage expectantly** with twice-weekly NSTs and AFIs, awaiting spontaneous labor.

5. **Take interventions for meconium-stained amniotic fluid** identified in labor.
   a. **Prior to delivery.** Begin gravity infusion of normal saline through an intrauterine catheter (amnioinfusion) to dilute the meconium.
   b. **After delivery of the fetal head.** Suction meconium from the nose and pharynx of the fetus to prevent aspiration.
   c. **After delivery of the entire fetus** but before the first neonatal breath. Aspirate neonatal tracheal meconium using a laryngoscope.

Clinical Situation 11–1

Basic Case: A 25-year-old multigravida comes to the maternity unit stating that fluid gushed from her vagina 2 hours ago.

Patient Snapshot	Intervention	Clinical Pearls
Her perineum appears moist to gross inspection. Nitrazine paper applied to the perineum turns blue.	Perform a speculum exam to rule out urinary incontinence.	**Alkaline urine** (common in pregnancy) can turn pH- sensitive nitrazine paper blue.
➡ 20 minutes later: Speculum exam shows posterior fornix fluid that turns nitrazine paper blue, and an air-dried glass slide makes a ferning pattern.	Confirm gestational age.	The **speculum exam** confirms a diagnosis of **ruptured membranes.** Management depends on gestational age.
➡ **Scenario 1** Review of prenatal records and early sonograms confirms a gestational age of **17 weeks.**	Induce labor or manage at home.	At 17 weeks, the likelihood of perinatal survival is extremely low. **Pulmonary hypoplasia** risk is high.
➡ **Scenario 2** Review of prenatal records and early sonograms confirms a gestational age of **27 weeks.**	Use conservative management in hospital. Give maternal steroids and antibiotics.	Risks of prematurity from 25 to 35 weeks are greater than risks of in utero infection. **"Leave baby in."** Take cultures and give prophylactic antibiotics and betamethasone.
➡ **Scenario 3** Review of her prenatal records and early sonograms confirms a gestational age of **37 weeks.**	Induce labor promptly.	Risks of in utero infection after 35 weeks are greater than risks of delivery. **"Get baby out."**
Rupture of membranes is confirmed. The uterus is tender to palpation. Vital signs are temperature, 102°F; blood pressure, 130/75 mm Hg; heart rate, 100 beats/min; and respirations, 22/min.	Induce labor; start broad-spectrum antibiotics.	**Fever** is a high predictor of **chorioamnionitis. At any gestational age, deliver the infant.** Organisms are probably normal genital flora. Treat for anaerobes and aerobes.
➡ Regular UCs are noted. Her cervix is 3 cm dilated.	Do not use tocolysis.	**Premature labor** in the presence of PROM is presumptive evidence of chorioamnionitis. Labor should not be stopped.

PROM = premature rupture of membranes   UC = uterine contraction

Clinical Situation 11–2

Basic Case: A 24-year-old primigravida at 29 weeks' gestation is under observation in the maternity unit. She complains of UCs every 5–7 minutes. The electronic fetal monitoring tracing is reassuring.

Patient Snapshot	Intervention	Clinical Pearls
Her cervix is closed, long, posterior, and firm. The head is high and unengaged.	Use conservative management.	**False labor** is defined as UCs without cervical dilation or effacement. Tocolytic agents are not used without evidence of cervical change.
➡ 2 weeks later: at 31 weeks, she returns with persistent UCs. Now her cervix is 2 cm dilated, 50% effaced.	Rule out contraindications for tocolysis.	With cervical change, now **true labor** can be diagnosed. Ensure that the fetus and mother will benefit from prolonging the pregnancy.
➡ 3 hours later: UCs continue. Mother and fetus are stable, and membranes are intact. There are no contraindications to tocolysis.	Start IV MgSO$_4$ loading dose, then continuous infusion.	**Tocolysis** can be initiated with MgSO$_4$, ritodrine, or nifedipine. Give mother betamethasone to induce fetal pulmonary maturity.
➡ 1 hour later: UCs are 3/hour. Cervical exam shows no change. Respirations have decreased from 20/min to 5/min.	Stop MgSO$_4$. Administer antidote.	**Respiratory depression** is a known side effect of magnesium toxicity. Administer IV calcium gluconate as antidote for Mg toxicity.
➡ 2 days later: UCs continue. She complains of vaginal fluid leakage. Speculum exam confirms that membranes have ruptured. An NST is reactive.	Do not give tocolytics. Use conservative management as long as fetal status is stable.	With membranes ruptured, early **chorioamnionitis** could be a cause of labor. Tocolysis is now contraindicated.
Her cervix is 2 cm dilated, 50% effaced. However, her uterus is tender and she has a temperature of 102°F.	Do not give tocolytics. Start broad-spectrum antibiotics and move toward delivery.	With evidence of **chorioamnionitis,** management is therapeutic antibiotics and initiation of delivery. Tocolytic agents are contraindicated.
Her cervix is 8 cm dilated, completely effaced, 0 station.	Use conservative management. Allow vaginal delivery.	With **advanced dilation,** the likelihood of successful tocolysis is so low that the risk to the mother is not justified.

IV = intravenous   NST = nonstress test   UC = uterine contraction

Clinical Situation 11–3

Basic Case: A 33-year-old multigravida is now 42 0/7 weeks gestation by dates.

Patient Snapshot	Intervention	Clinical Pearls
The gestational age is calculated using the LMP and a pregnancy wheel. However, she has **21-day menstrual cycles.**	Subtract 7 days from the EDD calculated by LMP.	Calculations of due date based on LMP assume a 28-day cycle. With known 21-day cycles, **ovulation** would have occurred on **day 7,** not day 14.
The gestational age is calculated using the LMP and a pregnancy wheel. However, she has **35-day menstrual cycles.**	Add 7 days to the EDD calculated by LMP.	Calculations of due date based on LMP assume a 28-day cycle. With known 35-day cycles, **ovulation** would have occurred on **day 21,** not day 14.
Her first sonogram showed a 10-week pregnancy. This differed by 7 days from the gestational age calculated by using her LMP.	Use sonogram due date, not LMP due date.	The accuracy of gestational age by < 12-week sonogram is ± 5 days. If the LMP gestational age is within 5 days of sonogram gestational age, use LMP gestational age. If it differs by more than 5 days, **use sonogram gestational age.**
Her first sonogram showed a 15-week pregnancy. This differed by 5 days from the gestational age calculated by using her LMP.	Use LMP due date, not sonogram due date.	The accuracy of gestational age by 12–18-week sonogram is ± 7 days. If the LMP gestational age is within 7 days of sonogram gestational age, **use LMP gestational age.** If it differs by more than 7 days, use sonogram gestational age.

EDD = estimated due date   LMP = last menstrual period

Clinical Situation 11–4

Basic Case: A 33-year-old multigravida is now 42 0/7 weeks gestation by dates. She just moved to the area and is transferring her obstetric care to you.

Patient Snapshot	Intervention	Clinical Pearls
She presents for a prenatal visit.	Establish how sure her dates are.	Management depends on your degree of **confidence** that she is **actually 2 weeks past her true due date.**
1 hour later: review of prenatal records and early sonogram shows her **dates are sure.** Her cervix is 3 cm dilated, 1-cm long, soft, −1 station.	Induce labor with AROM or oxytocin.	**Initiate delivery** with dates sure and favorable cervix. There is no benefit to either mother or ... the pregnancy.
Review of prenatal records and early sonogram shows her **dates are sure.** Her cervix is long, closed, firm, posterior.	Induce labor with PGE$_2$ or initiate fetal testing and await labor.	**PGE$_2$** can be used to ripen the cervix and induce labor with dates sure with unfavorable cervix. Otherwise, perform twice-weekly **NSTs and AFIs** while awaiting spontaneous labor.
Review of prenatal records shows her **dates are unsure.** No early sonogram was performed.	Perform twice-weekly NSTs and AFIs, and await labor.	Because gestational age is unsure, **conservative management is appropriate** as long as fetal well-being is assured.
2 days later: NST is reactive, but **AFI is 3.0 cm.**	Induce labor.	The low AFI is suggestive of **chronic placental insufficiency,** placing the fetus at risk. Delivery is indicated.
8 hours later: Labor is being induced, and she is 5 cm dilated. Membranes have just ruptured, with minimal AF seen. EFM shows **variable decelerations.**	Start amnioinfusion therapy.	Saline infused into the uterus provides a **pseudoamniotic fluid** that cushions the umbilical cord, preventing compression.
2 hours later: She is now 7 cm dilated, and **thick meconium** is noted.	Take steps to prevent meconium aspiration syndrome.	Preventive measures include **amnioinfusion** in labor, **suctioning** fetal nares and pharynx on perineum, and **tracheal aspiration** of any meconium seen near the vocal cords.

AFI = amniotic fluid index   EDD = estimated due date   LMP = last menstrual period
AROM = artificial rupture of membranes   EFM = electronic fetal monitoring   NST = nonstress test

12

Postpartum Issues

I. NORMAL PUERPERIUM

A. Overview

1. Definition. The puerperium is the time required for reversal of the changes of pregnancy.

2. Time required. The **time necessary for reversal** varies by organ system involved.
   a. By the end of the first day. Estradiol has fallen to normal, human placental lactogen (hPL) is undetectable, lung volumes are normal, and uterine weight is 1000 g.
   b. By the end of the first week. Fatty acid, glucose, and insulin values are normal, and uterine weight is 500 g.
   c. By the end of the first month. Total blood volume and peripheral vascular resistance are normal, human chorionic gonadotropin (hCG) is undetectable, and uterine weight is 100 g.
   d. By the end of the third month. Cholesterol and triglyceride values are normal, kidneys and ureters have normalized, and 10 L of body fluid have been lost.

B. Normal postpartum conditions. Postpartum changes relate to the gastrointestinal (GI), urinary, and reproductive tracts, which undergo significant changes during pregnancy.

1. Vaginal flow. Bright red bleeding is not normal. Normal **lochia,** the shedding of the decidual superficial layers, is managed conservatively.
   a. Lochia **rubra** (red) is seen in the first few days.
   b. Lochia **serosa** (pinkish-yellow) is seen up to the second week.
   c. Lochia **alba** (white) is seen after the second week.

2. Lower midline cramping. Mild analgesics may relieve normal postpartum uterine contractions.

3. Episiotomy pain. Ice packs in the first 24 hours help reduce perineal edema, and a heat lamp then enhances tissue fluid mobilization.

4. Constipation. Oral hydration should be encouraged, and stool softeners should be provided.

5. Hemorrhoids. The stool should be kept soft, and stool softeners (dioctyl sulfosuccinyl) and sitz baths should be provided.

6. Postvoid residual volume (> 250 ml). A hypotonic bladder may need time to recover. A cholinergic agonist (bethanechol 10 mg PO q6hr) should be tried. Intermittent catheterization or a continuous indwelling catheter may be needed.

7. **Mother is Rh-negative; neonate is Rh-positive.** Rh(D) isoimmunization can be prevented with the intramuscular (IM) administration of RhoGAM within 72 hours.

8. **Mother is rubella-susceptible.** Live attenuated rubella vaccine **should be administered intramuscularly.** Breastfeeding is permissible, but pregnancy should be avoided for 1 month.

C. **Contraceptive decision-making. Breastfeeding** may be associated with anovulation for up to 3 months, but barrier methods provide safe back-up contraception.

1. **Vaginal diaphragm.** Vaginal dimensions may change after pregnancy. Diaphragm refitting should be delayed for 6 weeks to allow postpartum vaginal involution.

2. **Progestin-only contraception.** This contraceptive method can be used in lactating women because milk yield is not affected. Oral pills, depomedroxyprogesterone acetate (Depo-Provera), or Norplant may be started immediately postpartum.

3. **Combination oral contraception.** The estrogen component can decrease milk yield, so this method should be avoided in lactating women. Combination oral contraception should be deferred in nonlactating women until postpartum week 3 to allow reversal of the hypercoagulable state of pregnancy.

4. **Intrauterine device (IUD).** Placement should be deferred until 6 weeks after delivery because of high expulsion rates if IUD placement occurs immediately postdelivery.

D. **Emotional response.** Normal parturients experience joy and happiness on seeing their newborn infants. Abnormal emotional responses, which have high recurrence rates, are causes for concern.

1. **Impaired mother–infant bonding** is more common when neonates are in the neonatal intensive care unit or if mothers perceive a lack of social support.
   a. **Finding:** no maternal interest in infants (e.g., mothers do not name their infants and do not want to see them)
   b. **Management:** psychosocial evaluation and intervention

2. **Postpartum blues** occur in over 50% of women within 2 weeks of delivery.
   a. **Findings:** tearfulness, wide mood swings, feelings of inadequacy but caring for themselves and their infants
   b. **Management:** reassurance and support (no medications are necessary)

3. **Postpartum depression** occurs in over 10% of women within 6 weeks of delivery.
   a. **Findings:** absence of tearfulness but feelings of despair, hopelessness, and anxiety; neglect care of themselves and their infants
   b. **Management:** psychotherapy and antidepressants

4. **Postpartum psychosis** (rare) occurs within 3 weeks of delivery.
   a. **Findings:** impairment of reality perception with hallucinations and delusions
   b. **Management:** hospitalization, antipsychotics, and psychotherapy

II. POSTPARTUM HEMORRHAGE (PPH)

A. **Definition.** PPH involves loss of over 500 ml (vaginal delivery) or 1000 ml (cesarean section) of blood in the first 24 hours postpartum.

B. **Etiology and risk factors**

1. **Uterine atony [*most common* overall cause (50%)].** **Risk factors** include rapid or protracted labor (*most common*); infected uterus; $MgSO_4$; and overdistended uterus (macrosomia, twins, polyhydramnios).

    2. **Genital laceration (20%). Risk factors** include uncontrolled vaginal delivery (*most common*)**,** large-sized infant, and use of forceps or vacuum extraction.

    3. **Retained placenta (10%). Risk factors** include noncontracted uterus (*most common*)**,** accessory placental lobe, and placenta accreta.

    4. **Disseminated intravascular coagulation (DIC) [rare]. Risk factors** include abruptio placentae (*most common*)**,** severe preeclampsia, amniotic fluid embolism, and fetal demise.

    5. **Uterine inversion (rare). Risk factors** include myometrial weakness (*most common*) and previous uterine inversion.

C. **Clinical findings and management (Table 12–1)**

D. **Additional treatment. If there is no response to conservative measures,** exploratory laparotomy may be required to ligate the uterine or internal iliac arteries bilaterally. Rarely, total hysterectomy may be necessary.

Table 12–1
Clinical Aspects of Postpartum Hemorrhage (PPH)

Causal Condition	Clinical Findings	Management
Uterine atony (50%)	• Soft uterus (i.e., like dough) that is palpable above the umbilicus	• Uterine massage • Oxytocin (20 U IV in 1000 ml saline) • Methylergonovine (0.2 IM) • Carboprost (250 μg IM)
Genital laceration (20%)	• Contracted uterus • Visualizable vaginal, cervical, or vulvar lacerations	• Thorough examination followed by prompt suturing under adequate anesthesia
Retained placenta (10%)	• Missing cotyledon on the maternal placental surface or extension of the vessels out to the membranes beyond the placental disk on the fetal surface • Failure of the placenta to separate	• Manual uterine exploration • Ultrasound-guided uterine curettage
Disseminated intravascular coagulation (DIC) [rare]	• Generalized bleeding or oozing in the presence of a contracted uterus	• Removal from the uterus of all POCs • Intensive care support • Selected blood product replacement [red blood cells (RBCs), platelets, fresh frozen plasma]
Uterine inversion (rare)	• Failure to palpate the uterus abdominally • Dark, beefy-appearing bleeding mass in the vagina or at the introitus	• Uterine replacement by elevating vaginal forces and lifting the uterus upward, followed by IV oxytocin

IV = intravenous   POC = products of conception   RBC = red blood cell
IM = intramuscular

III. POSTPARTUM FEVER

A. Definition. Temperatures in postpartum fever reach 100.4°F (38.0°C) or higher. The fevers occur on any two of the first 10 days postpartum, exclusive of the first 24 hours.

B. Incidence. Postpartum fever occurs after vaginal delivery in 1% of cases but after cesarean delivery in up to 30% of cases.

C. Bacterial pathogenesis. Ascending polymicrobial genital flora may be anaerobic, aerobic, gram-negative, or gram-positive.

D. Etiology and risk factors. Causes (listed in order of decreasing frequency) include endometritis *(most common),* urinary tract infection (UTI), pneumonia/atelectasis, wound infection, and septic pelvis thrombophlebitis. Specific risk factors for each etiologic condition are listed in order of the postpartum day (PPD) on which the condition generally occurs **(Chart 12–1).**

   1. PPD 0: atelectasis (WIND). Risk factors include general anesthesia, cigarette smoking, and obstructive lung disease.

   2. PPD 1–2: UTI (WATER). Risk factors include multiple catheterizations during labor, multiple vaginal examinations during labor, and untreated bacteriuria.

   3. PPD 2–3: endometritis (WOMB: *most common* **cause** of postpartum fever). **Risk factors** include **emergency cesarean section, prolonged membrane rupture, prolonged labor,** and multiple vaginal examinations during labor.

   4. PPD 4–5: wound infection (WOUND). Risk factors include **emergency cesarean section, prolonged membrane rupture, prolonged labor,** and multiple vaginal examinations during labor.

Postpartum Fever by Postpartum Day

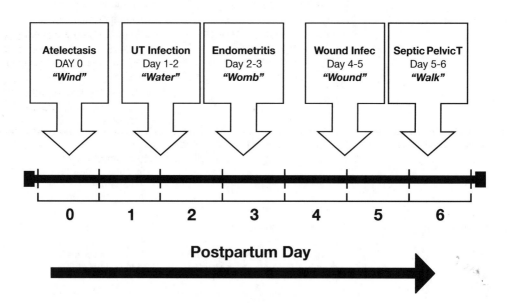

Chart 12–1.

5. PPD 5–6: septic pelvic thrombophlebitis (WALK). **Risk factors** include emergency cesarean section, prolonged membrane rupture, prolonged labor, and difficult vaginal delivery.

6. PPD 7–21: mastitis. **Risk factors** include nipple trauma from breastfeeding.

E. Clinical findings and management (Table 12–2)

Table 12–2
Clinical Aspects of Postpartum Fever

PPD	Causal Condition	Clinical Findings	Management
0	**Atelectasis (WIND)**	• Mild-to-moderate fever • No changes or mild rales on chest auscultation	• Pulmonary exercises • Ambulation
1–2	**Urinary tract infection (WATER)**	• High fever • Malaise • CVA tenderness • Positive urine culture	• Antibiotics as per urine culture sensitivity (single-agent: cephalosporin 1–2 g PO q6hr)
2–3	**Endometritis (WOMB)**	• Moderate fever • Exquisite uterine tenderness • Minimal abdominal findings	• Multiple-agent IV antibiotics to cover polymicrobial organisms: clindamycin 900 mg q8hr, gentamicin 500 mg every day • Addition of ampicillin 1–2 g IV q6hr if no response • No cultures are necessary
4–5	**Wound infection (WOUND)**	• Persistent spiking fever despite antibiotics • Wound erythema or fluctuance • Wound drainage	• Antibiotics for cellulitis • Open and drain wound • Saline-soaked packing twice a day • Secondary closure
5–6	**Septic pelvic thrombophlebitis (WALK)**	• Persistent wide fever swings despite antibiotics • Usually normal abdominal or pelvic exams	• IV heparin for 7–10 days at rates sufficient to prolong the PTT to double the baseline values
7–21	**Mastitis**	• Unilateral, localized erythema, edema, tenderness	• Antibiotics for cellulitis • Open and drain abscess if present

CVA = costovertebral angle   IV = intravenous   PPD = postpartum day
IM = intramuscular   PO = parenteral   PTT = partial thromboplastin time

Clinical Situation 12–1

Basic Case: A 36-year-old pregnant woman who smokes has undergone an emergency primary CS under general anesthesia. She was admitted with 18 hours of ruptured membranes and underwent IV oxytocin induction. Cervical dilation progressed to 8 cm but showed no further progress for 3 hours in spite of adequate labor.

Patient Snapshot	Intervention	Clinical Pearls
POD 0: 8 hours postop. Vital signs are temperature, 102°F; blood pressure, 130/75 mm Hg; heart rate, 100 beats/min; and respirations, 22/min. Lung fields are clear to auscultation.	Suggest ambulation and pulmonary exercises.	**Atelectasis** is seen within 24 hours. Risk factors are emergency CS with general anesthesia.
POD 2: She complains of urinary urgency. Her temperature is 102°F. She has mild right CVA tenderness.	Give single IV antibiotic after UA with CS.	**UTI** occurs on POD 1–2. Predisposing factors are indwelling Foley catheter and multiple vaginal exams.
POD 3: The urine culture shows no growth. Her temperature is 103°F. Exquisite uterine tenderness is present.	Give multiple IV antibiotics. No lochial culture is necessary.	**Endometritis** occurs on POD 2–3. Treat polymicrobial genital tract flora until the patient is afebrile for 48 hours.
POD 5: Spiking fevers to 102°F continue despite parenteral clindamycin and gentamicin. Abdominal wound purulent drainage is apparent.	Open the wound, placing saline-soaked packing.	**Wound infection** and **pelvic abscess** should be considered on POD 4–5. Pelvic imaging may be needed to identify abscess.
POD 6: "Picket-fence" fever is noted on IV antibiotics. No wound infection or abscess can be found. Worm-like masses can be palpated in the adnexae.	Order a baseline PTT, and then start IV heparin for 10–14 days.	**Septic pelvic thrombophlebitis** is often a diagnosis of exclusion. Fever resolution should be seen within 72 hours of IV heparin.

CS = cesarean section   POD = postoperative day   UA = urinalysis
CVA = costovertebral angle   PTT = partial thromboplastin time   UTI = urinary tract infection
IV = intravenous

13

Sexually Transmitted Disease

I. SEXUALLY TRANSMITTED DISEASES (STDs) WITH *PAINFUL* GENITAL ULCERS (Chart 13–1)

A. Herpes simplex virus (HSV)

1. **Etiology and epidemiology.** HSV, a DNA virus, is the *most common* **cause of genital ulcer disease.** HSV is one of the most contagious STDs, and transmission is by direct mucous membrane contact. Viremia occurs only with the primary infection, and the virus travels to the sensory root ganglia. An incurable latency is established. Recurrent disease occurs in only 30% of patients.

2. **Symptoms**
   a. **Primary herpes** is **systemic** with malaise; fever; adenopathy; and diffuse, exquisitely painful lesions.
   b. **Secondary herpes** is **localized** without systemic complaints. It may be activated by stress or menses and is preceded by prodromal paresthesias.

3. **Clinical examination.** Primary lesions consist of **clear vesicles** that develop at the site of exposure and spontaneously rupture, forming **shallow, painful ulcers with raised edges.** In recurrent disease, lesions are more localized, less severe, and of shorter duration.

4. **Laboratory tests.** Viral cultures are the most accurate for diagnosis. Monoclonal antibody or cytologic studies (multinucleated giant cells) are less reliable.

5. **Management.** Antiviral agents such as **acyclovir** (200 mg PO q4hr for 5 days) may decrease the duration and severity of symptoms. **Famciclovir** and **valacyclovir** are also used. **Valacyclovir has been shown to diminish the risk of sexual transmission of HSV by 50%.**

B. Chancroid

1. **Epidemiology.** *Haemophilus ducreyi,* a gram-negative bacterium, causes chancroid, a rare disease in the United States. The male:female ratio is 5:1. Chancroid ulcers can facilitate the transmission of human immunodeficiency virus (HIV).

2. **Symptoms.** The initial papule develops into a **pustule that becomes a painful ulcer** within 72 hours. The pustule occurs on the vulva and rarely on the vagina or cervix.

3. **Clinical examination.** A shallow, nonindurated, soft, **painful ulcer with a characteristically ragged edge** is seen. Tender inguinal adenopathy may develop.

STDs with Ulcers — *Comparison*

Chancroid *painful*	"Ragged soft" edge
LGV	"Groove" sign
Granuloma Inguinale	"Beefy red" ulcer
Syphilis	"Rolled hard" edge
Herpes *painful*	"Smooth" edge

Chart 13–1.

4. **Laboratory tests.** A positive culture confirms the diagnosis, but the organism is difficult to grow. Gram staining is not reliable. A clinical diagnosis is often made after syphilis has been ruled out.

5. **Management.** Azithromycin 1 g PO in a single dose or a single dose of **ceftriaxone** 250 mg IM.

II. SEXUALLY TRANSMITTED DISEASES (STDs) WITH *PAINLESS* GENITAL ULCERS

A. Syphilis

1. **Epidemiology.** *Treponema pallidum,* a motile anaerobic spirochete, causes syphilis. **Untreated primary syphilis** (with a **localized chancre**) spontaneously disappears and progresses to **secondary syphilis** (with **systemic manifestations**), which also spontaneously disappears and develops into **latent syphilis.** One-third of patients with latent disease progress to **tertiary disease.**

2. Symptoms
   a. **Primary syphilis** is **asymptomatic with a painless chancre** that resolves spontaneously.
   b. **Secondary syphilis,** the **result of hematogenous spirochetemia,** is characterized by fever, inguinal adenopathy, and **painless condylomata lata.**
   c. **Latent syphilis** is **asymptomatic.**
   d. **Tertiary syphilis** leads to numerous symptoms, which vary depending on the extent of **gumma involvement** of the central nervous system (CNS) as well as the cardiovascular and musculoskeletal systems.

3. Clinical examination
   a. In **primary syphilis,** the classic lesion is the **painless chancre** with an indurated rolled edge. This usually solitary lesion is found on the vulva, vagina, or cervix.
   b. In **secondary syphilis,** the classic lesion is the **condyloma lata,** an exophytic excrescence that may ulcerate. The **classic rash** of secondary syphilis is apparent as red macules and papules over the palms of the hands and feet **(money spots).**
   c. Findings in late **tertiary syphilis** may mimic many diseases, including optic atrophy, tabes dorsalis, generalized paresis, aortic aneurysm, and gummas of the skin and bones.

4. **Laboratory tests.** *T. pallidum*, an extremely thin spirochete, can be seen only with a darkfield microscope.
   a. **Screening for *T. pallidum*.** Nonspecific serologic tests such as the **Venereal Disease Research Laboratory (VDRL) test** or the **rapid plasma reagin (RPR) test** can be used to follow the treatment course. **False-positive results** frequently occur with autoimmune diseases such as lupus and with viral infections.
   b. **Confirmation of diagnosis.** A treponema-specific test such as a **fluorescent titer antibody absorption (FTA-ABS)** or **microhemagglutination assay for antibodies to *T. pallidum* (MHA-TP)** is used.

5. **Management. Penicillin is the drug of choice.** A single dose of **benzathine penicillin G** (2.4 million U IM) is given for primary, secondary, and early latent disease.
   a. For **penicillin-allergic nonpregnant patients, tetracycline** 500 mg PO q6hr for 2 weeks is used.
   b. For **penicillin-allergic pregnant patients, penicillin** with an **oral desensitization schedule** is used.

B. **Lymphogranuloma venereum (LGV)**

   1. **Epidemiology.** The L serotype of **Chlamydia trachomatis** causes this chronic lymphatic infection. LGV, which has a male:female ratio of 5:1, is rare in the United States.

   2. Symptoms
      a. **Subclinical primary infection** is common, with a painless vulvar ulcer that spontaneously heals.
      b. The **secondary phase** is characterized by painful inguinal or **perirectal adenopathy.** If the condition is untreated, the enlarging nodes rupture, forming multiple draining abscesses or fistula.

   3. **Clinical examination.** The primary lesion is an elevated, painless, round or oval ulcer usually on the vulva, but possibly on the urethra, rectum, or cervix. The **classic clinical sign** is the double genitocrural fold, or **"groove sign,"** a depression between groups of tender, inflamed inguinal nodes.

   4. **Laboratory tests.** The diagnosis is established by a culture of pus aspirated from a tender lymph node or a positive monoclonal *Chlamydia* antibody test on the aspirated fluid. A compliment fixation antibody titer > 1:64 is indicative of an active infection.

   5. **Management. Doxycycline** 100 mg PO bid × 21 days or **erythromycin** base 500 mg PO q6hr for 3–6 weeks may be effective. Fluctuant nodes should be aspirated to prevent sinus formation.

C. **Granuloma inguinale (donovanosis)**

   1. **Epidemiology.** *Calymmatobacterium granulomatis,* a gram-negative bacterium, is the causative agent. This STD is rare in the United States. Because it is not very contagious, chronic exposure is necessary for disease spread.

2. Symptoms. The initial infection is asymptomatic, with only a localized nodule over which skin breakdown occurs. Multiple lesions can coalesce, and secondary infection is possible. Chronic scarring can lead to lymphatic obstruction.

3. Clinical examination. The initial lesion is a vulvar nodule that breaks down, forming a **painless, beefy red ulcer** with fresh granulation tissue. Lymphatic obstruction can result in marked vulvar enlargement.

4. Laboratory test. Diagnosis is confirmed by the identification of **Donovan bodies** in smears and ulcer specimens.

5. Management. Doxycycline 100 mg PO bid × 21 days or trimethoprim sulfamethaxazole one double-strength tablet PO bid × 21 days. If medical therapy fails, surgical excision is required.

III. SEXUALLY TRANSMITTED DISEASES (STDs) *WITHOUT* GENITAL ULCERS

A. Condyloma acuminatum

1. Epidemiology. Human papilloma virus (HPV), the etiologic agent, **causes the *most common*** overall STD and the *most common* viral STD. HPV is highly infectious and can be transmitted by both microscopic and macroscopic lesions. **HPV subtypes 16 and 18** are associated with female genital tract malignancies. Predisposing factors include immunosuppression, diabetes, pregnancy, and local trauma.

2. Symptoms. HPV is **subclinical** in **70% of women.** Pain, odor, or bleeding may occur when the condylomata become large or infected.

3. Clinical examination. Initially, lesions are found in the vestibule, but eventually, they **spread by autoinoculation** to the vagina, cervix, urethra, bladder, and rectum. Lesions vary in size and may be single or in clusters. **Macroscopic pedunculated warts** are noted on moist perineal skin in **only 30% of infected women.**

4. Laboratory test. Biopsy is usually unnecessary, because **usually the diagnosis is obvious clinically.** However, questionable lesions should be biopsied.

5. Management. Treatment is directed only at clinical lesions. Small lesions are treated topically with **podophyllin, trichloroacetic acid,** or **imiquimod.** Larger lesions are ablated with cryotherapy, laser vaporization, or surgical excision. No effective systemic therapy is available.

B. Chlamydia

1. Epidemiology. *Chlamydia trachomatis,* an obligate intracellular bacterium, is the *most common* cause of most cases of mucopurulent cervicitis. **Chlamydial infection is the *most common* bacterial STD in women.**

  a. Vertical transmission to newborns may result in inclusion **conjunctivitis** and **otitis media.**

  b. Women who take oral contraceptives show a twofold increase in positive endocervical cultures for **C. *trachomatis*** but no increase in pelvic inflammatory disease (PID).

  c. Risk factors include **sexual activity at age < 20 years,** multiple sexual partners, lower socioeconomic status, and other STDs.

2. Symptoms. Most chlamydial cervical infections, and even salpingitis, are **asymptomatic.** Urethritis and lower abdominal or pelvic pain may be seen.

3. Clinical examination. Chlamydia infects only the endocervical and endotubal mucosa without involving the squamous epithelium. **Mucopurulent cervical discharge** is frequently noted on speculum examination. Urethral and cervical motion tenderness may be apparent.

4. Laboratory tests. In the past, tissue culture was the diagnostic gold standard. Now, polymerase chain reaction (PCR) and DNA probe assays, which are equivalent in sensitivity and specificity, are used.

5. Management. Azithromycin 1 g PO in a single dose is effective or **doxycyline** 100 mg PO bid for 7 days. All sexual partners should receive the same treatment.

C. Gonorrhea

    1. Epidemiology. *Neisseria gonorrhoeae,* a gram-negative diplococcal bacterium, is the causative organism.

        a. Sites of infection include the cervix, anal canal, urethra, oropharynx, and Bartholin's glands.

        b. Vertical transmission may result in neonatal conjunctivitis.

        c. Disseminated infection may occur in 1% of cases, causing tenosynovitis, dermatitis, pericarditis, and meningitis.

    2. Symptoms. Early infections may be **asymptomatic.**

        a. Lower genital **tract** involvement may lead to only vulvovaginal discharge, itching and burning with dysuria, or rectal discomfort.

        b. Upper genital **tract** involvement may result in PID, leading to diffuse bilateral pelvic or abdominal pain with nausea, vomiting, and fever.

    3. Clinical examination

        a. Mucopurulent cervical discharge is frequently noted on speculum examination. **Cervical motion tenderness** may be seen.

        b. Vulvovaginitis is not seen in estrogenized adults but may develop with invasion of nonkeratinized squamous epithelium in prepubertal children or postmenopausal women.

        c. Bartholin's abscess manifests as a painful, erythematous mass at the introitus when the duct to an infected gland is obstructed. If healing occurs but the abscess is not drained, a nontender **Bartholin's cyst** results.

    4. Laboratory test. The **diagnostic standard is culture** of endocervical mucus and a rectal swab directly onto Thayer-Martin media.

    5. Management

        a. Patients infected with *N. gonorrhea* are often coinfected with *C. trachomatis.* Therefore routine dual therapy for both should be given without testing for chlamydia.

        b. Uncomplicated cervicitis is treated with cefixime 400 mg PO in a single dose, plus azithromycin 1 g PO in a single dose.

        c. Bartholin's abscess is treated with antibiotics, followed by incision and placement of a small rubber catheter, allowing the abscess to continue draining while healing.

D. Hepatitis B virus (HBV)

    1. Epidemiology

        a. HBV, which is caused by a DNA hepadnavirus, is **transmitted by body fluids** (e.g., blood, semen, vaginal or oral secretions, breast milk). **It is the only STD that can be prevented by immunization.**

        b. Carrier rates approach 35% in Asia and Africa. Mother–infant transmission causes 40% of all chronic HBV infections.

    2. Symptoms. Most HBV infections are **asymptomatic.** Acute and chronic HBV can result in right upper quadrant pain and lethargy, depending on the infection severity.

3. Clinical examination. In acute hepatitis, right upper quadrant tenderness may be present.

4. Laboratory tests. Hepatitis B surface antigen (HBsAg) is the *most common screening marker* that identifies carrier status. **Hepatitis B e antigen (HBeAg)** is an accurate predictor of viral replication and infectivity. **Liver enzyme elevation** with elevated serum bilirubin indicates active or chronic disease.

5. Management. No specific therapy is used for most acute hepatitis. Alpha interferon or lamivudine may be given in cases with severe liver enzyme elevation. Carriers of HBsAg should be screened for liver involvement.

6. Prevention. Vaccination should be offered to household members and sexual contacts of patients with HBsAg. This should include **passive immunization** with hepatitis B immune globulin and **active immunization** with hepatitis B killed virus vaccine.

E. Human immunodeficiency virus (HIV)

1. Epidemiology
   a. The RNA retrovirus that causes HIV is the etiologic agent responsible for **acquired immunodeficiency syndrome (AIDS).** HIV is **transmitted by body fluids.**
   b. HIV has a predilection for cells of the immune system. Over a period of years, as the virus incorporates itself into the genome of host cells, declining cell-mediated immunity results in opportunistic infections that eventually kill the infected host.

2. Symptoms
   a. The initial infection is asymptomatic; only the **acute viral syndrome** is noted within the first few weeks.
   b. After a latent period of 5–7 years, falling CD4 helper T cell counts are reflected in **AIDS-related complex,** night sweats, malaise, diarrhea, weight loss, and unusual recurrent opportunistic infections.

3. Clinical examination. The early stages of HIV have no distinct physical findings.
   a. With deteriorating immunity, symptoms and signs of **opportunistic diseases** such as tuberculosis, *Pneumocystis carinii* pneumonia, toxoplasmosis, cytomegalovirus (CMV), and HSV may be evident.
   b. The **frequency of cervical dysplasia and carcinoma is higher** in HIV-positive women. AIDS is diagnosed in HIV-positive women with cervical carcinoma.

4. Laboratory tests
   a. Screening entails an **enzyme-linked immunosorbent assay (ELISA)** that checks for the presence of antibodies against HIV.
   b. Confirmation following persistently positive ELISA results is a positive **Western blot** test. The most specific test is a **PCR test** for HIV RNA.

5. Management
   a. Zidovudine, a reverse transcriptase inhibitor, is the most widely used antiviral agent. This agent is recommended for asymptomatic women with CD4 counts below 500/mm^3.
   b. Protease inhibitors are added as part of multiple-drug therapy in symptomatic HIV disease.

14

Pelvic Inflammatory Disease

I. ACUTE SALPINGO-OOPHORITIS. This condition is the *most common* **presentation of pelvic inflammatory disease (PID),** a disorder that involves the upper genital tract, specifically the oviducts and ovaries. After only one episode of untreated PID, the risk of infertility from tubal adhesions is 15%.

A. Etiology

  1. *Chlamydia trachomatis,* which also causes the *most common* **sexually transmitted disease (STD) of bacterial origin,** is the *most common* **pathogen.** *Neisseria gonorrhoeae* also causes PID.

  2. These pathogens ascend from the lower genital tract (vagina, cervix) to the upper genital tract (endosalpingeal mucosa, ovaries). The **likelihood of ascending infection is increased** by the loss of the protective barrier of cervical mucus **at the time of menses (Chart 14–1).**

B. Risk factors

  1. **Increased risk: age < 20 years,** multiple sexual partners, prior PID, vaginal douching

  2. **Decreased risk:** older age, monogamy, barrier contraception, steroid contraception

C. **Symptoms. Bilateral abdominal-pelvic pain** is characteristic, but the degree is variable depending on the extent of infection. Onset may be gradual or sudden. Nonspecific symptoms such as pelvic pressure or back pain that radiates down the legs may be present. Nausea and vomiting may be reported with severe infections.

D. **Clinical examination. Mucopurulent cervical discharge, cervical motion tenderness,** and **bilateral adnexal tenderness** are characteristic. Low-grade fever with tachycardia is common, but high fevers can occur. **Abdominal findings (e.g., tenderness, rebound, ileus) are bilateral** and vary with degree of peritoneal involvement.

E. **Diagnostic findings. Cervical cultures** are positive for the pathogenic organisms. In addition, the **white blood cell (WBC) count** and **erythrocyte sedimentation rate (ESR)** are elevated. **Sonography** is not usually helpful, because it does not reveal inflammatory changes. **Laparoscopy** is diagnostic in visualizing acute inflammation of the oviducts. **Culdocentesis** reveals pus in the cul-de-sac if gross suppurative purulence is present.

F. **Differential diagnosis.** Any cause of pelvic pain, including adnexal torsion, ectopic pregnancy, endometriosis, appendicitis, diverticulitis, regional ileitis, and ulcerative colitis, should be considered.

  1. **Ectopic pregnancy should be ruled out** with β-human chorionic gonadotropin (β-hCG) testing.

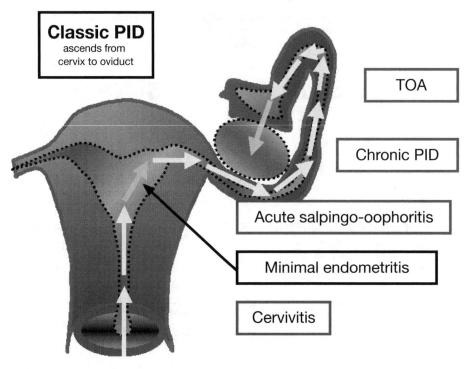

Chart 14–1.

2. **Gastrointestinal (GI) and urinary tract causes of pain** (e.g., appendicitis, pyelonephritis) **should be ruled out.**

G. Management. Therapy may be outpatient or inpatient, depending on the severity of infection and the likelihood of infertility from inadequate treatment.

    1. **Inpatient treatment. Patients should be hospitalized if any of the following criteria are present:** evidence of pelvic abscess, temperature > 102.2°F (39°C), inability to follow or tolerate oral therapy, pregnancy, outpatient treatment failure, severe illness, or uncertain diagnosis. **Inpatient antibiotic therapy** involves parenteral **cefoxitin** (2 g IV q6hr) + **doxycycline** (100 mg IV or PO q12hr) *or* **clindamycin** (900 mg IV q8hr) + **gentamicin** (1.5 mg/kg IV q8hr).

    2. **Outpatient treatment. Outpatient antibiotic therapy** involves **cefoxitin** [2 g IM (single dose)] with **probenecid** (1 g PO) + **doxycycline** (100 mg PO bid for 14 days).

II. CHRONIC PELVIC INFLAMMATORY DISEASE (PID)

A. Etiology. Chronic PID arises from untreated or inadequately treated acute salpingo-oophoritis that resolved spontaneously but resulted in the formation of diffuse **intraperitoneal adhesions** involving the uterus, oviducts, ovaries, bowel, and omentum. **No active inflammation is present.**

B. Symptoms. All symptoms are the consequences of **pelvic adhesions. Bilateral chronic abdominal-pelvic pain** is characteristic. Other symptoms (e.g., infertility, pain with intercourse, previous ectopic pregnancy) are the consequence of pelvic adhesions.

C. Clinical examination. No fever is present. However, **bilateral abdominal-cervical-adnexal tenderness** is evident. One or more adnexal masses may be found if a hydrosalpinx is present. **Mucopurulent cervical discharge is absent.**

D. Diagnostic findings. Cervical cultures are negative. **WBC count** and the **ESR** are within normal limits. Sonography may show a dilated hydrosalpinx. **Laparoscopy is definitive for visualizing pelvic adhesions.**

E. Differential diagnosis. Any cause of pelvic pain, including adnexal torsion, ectopic pregnancy, endometriosis, appendicitis, diverticulitis, regional ileitis, and ulcerative colitis, should be considered.

F. Management. Because no active infectious process is present, **antibiotics are not indicated.** Analgesics and narcotics provide only temporary respite due to development of medication tolerance. **Lysis of adhesions** seldom yields permanent pain relief. Complete **pelvic clean-out** [total abdominal hysterectomy and bilateral salpingo-oophorectomy (TAH-BSO)] may provide the only chance for pain eradication.

III. TUBO-OVARIAN ABSCESS (TOA)

A. Etiology. A TOA arises from untreated or inadequately treated acute salpingo-oophoritis that fails to resolve but instead forms a **purulent inflammatory mass** involving the uterus, oviducts, ovaries, bowel, and omentum.

B. Symptoms. Severe **bilateral abdominal-pelvic pain** is present. Nausea and vomiting are common because of bowel involvement.

C. Clinical examination. Sepsis is usually apparent. High fever [temperature up to 103°F (39.4°C)] is frequent.

    1. Peritoneal signs such as abdominal guarding, ileus, and rigidity with rebound tenderness are characteristic.

    2. Pelvic examination signs include mucopurulent cervical discharge. Exquisite cervical motion and rectal tenderness, with **bilateral, tender adnexal masses** are typical.

D. Diagnostic findings. Cervical cultures are positive for pathogenic organisms (*C. trachomatis, N. gonorrhoeae*). Anaerobic secondary invaders (*Bacteroides* sp.) are frequent. The **WBC count** and **ESR** are markedly elevated. **Sonography** shows bilateral adnexal masses.

E. Differential diagnosis. Any cause of severe abdominal-pelvic pain, including septic abortion, periappendiceal abscess, adnexal torsion, ectopic pregnancy, and degenerating leiomyoma, should be considered.

F. Management

    1. Hospitalization is imperative. Parenteral **clindamycin** (900 mg IV q8hr) and **gentamicin** (500 mg IV q24hr) usually result in fever response and the beginning of TOA shrinkage within 48 hours.

    2. If medical antibiotic management does not lead to a clinical response, percutaneous **cul-de-sac drainage or emergency laparotomy may be necessary.**

Clinical Situation 14–1

Basic Case: A 22-year-old woman comes to the office complaining of bilateral lower abdominal tenderness. A urine β-hCG is negative.

Patient Snapshot	Intervention	Clinical Pearls
She has no fever but has mucopurulent cervical discharge, cervical motion tenderness, and bilateral adnexal tenderness.	Obtain cervical culture and then give **outpatient antibiotics.**	**Uncomplicated acute PID** is treated with IM cephalosporin (for gonorrhea) plus oral doxycyline (for chlamydia).
Her temperature is 102°F (38.9°C), with mucopurulent cervical discharge, cervical motion tenderness, and bilateral adnexal tenderness.	Obtain cervical cultures and then give **inpatient antibiotics.**	**Complicated acute PID** is treated with hospitalization and parenteral antibiotics.
Her temperature is 102°F (38.9°C), with mucopurulent cervical discharge, cervical motion tenderness, and **bilateral fluctuant adnexal masses.**	Obtain cervical cultures and then give **inpatient antibiotics.**	**TOA** is treated with hospitalization and parenteral antibiotics to cover anaerobes and gram negative organisms.
➔ 3 days later: She has been on parenteral clindamycin and gentamicin for > 48 hours, with no response to spiking fevers or size of the adnexal masses.	Perform **surgical drainage.**	Failed response to medical therapy calls for either **percutaneous cul-de-sac drainage** or **emergency laparotomy.**
She has a past history of PID. She has **no fever** and **no cervical discharge** but does have cervical motion tenderness and bilateral adnexal masses.	Perform **laparoscopy** to confirm adhesions. Mild analgesics.	Treatment for pain of **chronic PID** is often disappointing. TAH and BSO may be needed if the therapeutic reponse is unsatisfactory (remember to give ERT).

BSO = bilateral salpingo-oophorectomy   IM = intramuscular   TOA = tubo-ovarian abscess
ERT = estrogen replacement therapy   PID = pelvic inflammatory disease
hCG = human chorionic gonadotropin   TAH = total abdominal hysterectomy

15

Vaginal Discharge

I. DEFINITIONS

A. Physiologic discharge. This condition arises from normal desquamation of vaginal epithelium and estrogen-dominant cervical mucus.

1. **In appearance,** the discharge is thin and nonodorous, with a pH range of 3.5 to 4.5.

2. **Vaginal examination** reveals no vaginal erythema, edema, itching, or burning.

3. **Microbiologically,** facultative aerobes and anaerobes remain in low concentrations because of an acidic pH produced by the **dominant organism, lactobacillus.**

B. Vaginitis

1. This condition arises from an **inflammatory response,** resulting in symptoms of **itching, burning,** or pain, as well as signs of erythema and edema.

2. **Microscopic examination** of the discharge is positive for white blood cells (WBCs) and the causative organisms, usually *Candida* or *Trichomonas.*

C. Vaginosis

1. This condition arises from an alteration of normal flora, with a **marked decrease** in lactobacillus and a **significant increase** in aerobes and anaerobes.

2. There is no inflammatory response with erythema, edema, and WBCs. **Vaginal pH rises,** and **clue cells** are seen on saline preparations (epithelial cells studded with bacteria obscuring the cell borders). The current name for this disorder is **bacterial vaginosis (BV).**

II. BACTERIAL VAGINOSIS (BV). This condition is the *most common* cause of abnormal vaginal discharge in the United States **(Chart 15–1).**

A. Epidemiology. Anaerobic bacteria (*Bacteroides sp., Peptostreptococcus*) increase in concentration up to 1000-fold. Only 50% of patients are symptomatic.

B. Clinical findings

1. A thin, gray, adherent discharge with a **fishy, amine odor** is noted. **Vaginal pH is > 4.5.**

2. Minimal or no inflammatory changes are seen on examination.

3. Microscopic viewing of the discharge in saline shows minimal WBCs, with **clue cells** visible **(Figure 15–1).**

Change in Vaginal Flora with Bacterial Vaginosis

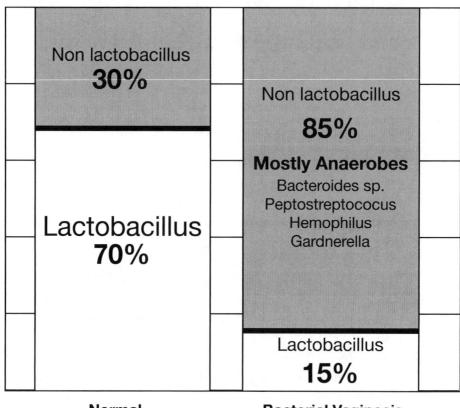

Non lactobacillus
30%

Lactobacillus
70%

Non lactobacillus
85%

Mostly Anaerobes
Bacteroides sp.
Peptostreptococus
Hemophilus
Gardnerella

Lactobacillus
15%

Normal   **Bacterial Vaginosis**

Chart 15–1.

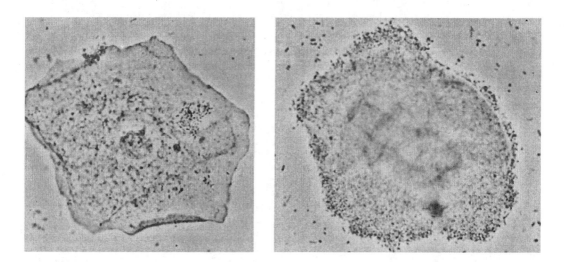

Figure 15–1.   Clue cells as seen in bacterial vaginosis. (From Vontver LA, Eschenback DA: The role of *Gardnerella vaginalis* in nonspecific vaginitis. *Clin Obstet Gynecol* 24:452–453, 1981.)

C. Management. Selected antibiotics are directed at anaerobic organisms. The sexual partner does not need treatment.

    1. Oral agents: metronidazole 500 mg or clindamycin bid for 7 days

    2. Vaginal agents: metronidazole gel (0.75%) or clindamycin cream (2%) bid for 7 days

III. CANDIDA VAGINITIS. This condition is the second *most common* cause of abnormal vaginal discharge.

  A. Epidemiology. Yeasts, especially *Candida albicans,* predominate. Yeast may be present in the vagina without symptoms. **Risk factors** include altered immunity [immunosuppression, human immunodeficiency virus (HIV)], uncontrolled diabetes, and systemic broad-spectrum antibiotics.

  B. Clinical findings

    1. A thick, curd-like, **white discharge** that has no odor is apparent. The **vaginal pH is < 4.5,** in the normal range.

    2. Vaginal erythema, edema, and tenderness are seen in symptomatic patients.

    3. Microscopic viewing of the discharge in saline shows abundant WBCs. Addition of 10% **potassium hydroxide (KOH)** solution reveals **pseudohyphae (Figure 15–2).**

  C. Management. The sexual partner does not require treatment unless symptomatic.

    1. Oral agents: fluconazole 150 mg (single dose)

    2. Vaginal agents: a variety of fungicidal "azole" creams (e.g., ticonazole, clotrimazole, miconazole, terconazole) for 3 to 7 days

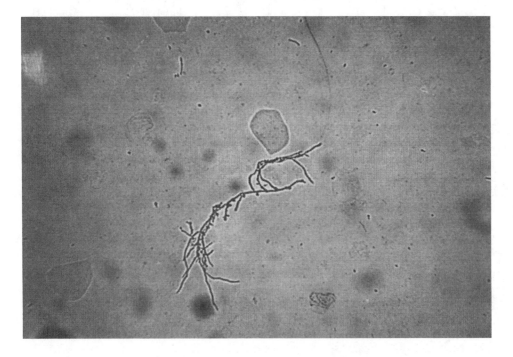

Figure 15–2.   Yeast cells and pseudomycelia in vaginal candidiasis as seen in a vaginal smear (a KOH prep). (From Merkus JMWM, Bisschop MPJM, Stolte LAM: *Obstet Gynecol Surv* 40:495, 1985. Copyright 1985 by Williams & Wilkins.)

IV. TRICHOMONAS VAGINITIS. This condition is the least common cause of abnormal vaginal discharge in the United States but the *most common* cause worldwide.

A. Epidemiology. The flagellated parasite *Trichomonas vaginalis* predominates. **Risk factors** include sexual transmission from the reproductive or urinary tracts.

B. Clinical findings

1. A profuse, frothy, **yellow-green, malodorous discharge** is noted. The **vaginal pH is > 4.5.**

2. Vaginal erythema, edema, and tenderness are seen in symptomatic patients.

3. Microscopic viewing of the discharge in saline shows abundant WBCs and the classic **motile flagellated parasites.**

C. Management. The sexual partner should receive oral treatment. The only effective agent is **metronidazole,** which can be administered either orally (500 mg bid for 7 days or a single 2 g dose).

Clinical Situation 15–1

Basic Case: A 23-year-old woman comes to the office concerned about vaginal discharge.

Patient Snapshot	Intervention	Clinical Pearls
She states that she has minimal discharge but that it has a **fishy odor.**	Obtain vaginal secretions for pH and "wet prep."	**BV seems the most likely diagnosis.** Look for vaginal pH ↑, positive "whiff" test, and wet prep with clue cells.
➥ On pelvic exam, no erythema or edema is seen. Vaginal pH is 5.5. Clue cells are apparent.	Give metronidazole or clindamycin orally or vaginally.	**BV is confirmed.** With BV, anaerobes are ↑ but lactobacillus are ↓. Treat the anaerobes. There is no need to treat the sexual partner.
She states she has profuse discharge associated with itching and pain.	Obtain vaginal secretions for pH and "wet prep."	The primary **differential diagnosis** is vaginitis due to yeast or trichomoniasis.
➥ On pelvic exam, erythema and edema are seen. Vaginal pH is 4.5. Pseudohyphae are apparent.	Give a single dose of fluconazole or vaginal "azole" creams for 3–7 days.	**Yeast vaginitis** is confirmed. There is no need to treat the sexual partner.
➥ On pelvic exam, erythema and edema are seen. Vaginal pH is 6.0. Motile flagellated organisms are apparent.	Give metronidazole orally.	**Trichomonas vaginitis** is confirmed. The sexual partner also must be treated. Warn the partner about an antabuse-like reaction with alcohol.

BV = bacterial vaginosis

16

Amenorrhea

I. OVERVIEW

A. Definitions

1. Primary amenorrhea
   a. No menses by **14 years of age** and **absence** of secondary sex characteristics
   b. No menses by age **16 years of age** with **presence** of secondary sex characteristics

2. Secondary amenorrhea
   a. No menses for **3 months** if previous menses were **regular**
   b. No menses for **6 months** if previous menses were **irregular**

B. Etiology

1. **HYPOgonadotropic causes [follicle-stimulating hormone (FSH) is low]** result from failure of either gonadotropin-releasing hormone (GnRH) secretion from the hypothalamus or FSH secretion from the anterior pituitary. Such conditions may involve central nervous system (CNS) tumors or be idiopathic.

2. **HYPERgonadotropic causes (FSH is high)** result from the absence (congenital or acquired) of ovarian follicles. Such conditions may include gonadal dysgenesis (45,X), ovarian follicle injury, or ovarian failure.

3. **Eugonadotropic causes (FSH is normal)** result from anovulation, uterine absence, endometrial scarring, cervical stenosis, intact hymen, or vaginal agenesis.

II. CLINICAL APPROACH TO PRIMARY AMENORRHEA. A thorough general and pelvic examination should first be performed.

A. Breasts are <u>ABSENT</u> but a uterus is <u>PRESENT</u>.

1. **Clinical findings.** Presence of breasts is a measure of endogenous estrogen. Absence of breasts must result from inadequate estrogen. **One of two conditions** may account for this.
   a. Follicles are not present in the ovary to produce estrogen.
   b. Follicles may be present, but because of hypothalamic or pituitary pathology, they are not being stimulated.

2. **Diagnosis. An FSH level and karyotype should be obtained.**
   a. The diagnosis is **gonadal dysgenesis,** the *most common* cause of primary amenorrhea (30%), if the FSH level is high and the karyotype is 45,X.
   b. The diagnosis is **hypothalamic-pituitary insufficiency** if the FSH level is low and the karyotype is normal.

3. Management. In both conditions, **estrogen** should be provided to stimulate secondary sexual development, along with **cyclic progestins** to prevent endometrial hyperplasia. If the FSH level is low, CNS imaging should be obtained to rule out a tumor.

B. Breasts are PRESENT but a uterus is ABSENT.

1. **Clinical findings.** Adequate estrogen must be produced by the gonads to stimulate breast development. The uterus is lacking in two groups of patients. In both cases, the oviducts, uterus, cervix, and proximal vagina are absent.
   a. Genetic females with idiopathic failure of müllerian development characterize **müllerian agenesis.**
   b. Genetic males with an absence of androgen receptors characterize **androgen insensitivity.** The Y chromosome has led to the production of müllerian inhibitory factor (MIF).

2. **Diagnosis. A testosterone level and karyotype should be obtained.**
   a. The diagnosis is **müllerian agenesis** if testosterone is at normal female levels and the karyotype is 46,XX (20% of cases of primary amenorrhea).
   b. The diagnosis is **androgen insensitivity** if testosterone is at high male levels and the karyotype is 46,XY (10% of cases of primary amenorrhea).

3. **Management.** In both conditions, a neovagina may need to be created. With androgen insensitivity, the undescended testes in the inguinal canal should be removed to prevent malignant changes. Estrogen replacement therapy (ERT) should then be initiated.

C. Breasts are PRESENT and a uterus is PRESENT. Differential diagnosis includes imperforate hymen, vaginal agenesis, or transverse vaginal septum. Pelvic examination will identify the cause. Otherwise an approach similar to that used with secondary amenorrhea can be taken with affected patients (see III).

III. CLINICAL APPROACH TO SECONDARY AMENORRHEA

A. A **β-human chorionic gonadotropin (β-hCG) level should be obtained** to rule out pregnancy, which is the *most common* cause of secondary amenorrhea.

B. A **progesterone challenge test (PCT) should be administered** (medroxyprogesterone acetate 10 mg PO for 7 days), and the occurrence of withdrawal bleeding should be noted.

1. The **PCT is positive** if any bleeding beyond a few drops occurs within 2–7 days. This always results from **anovulation.**
   a. Serum prolactin and thyroid-stimulating hormone (TSH) levels rule out a correctable cause of anovulation such as a pituitary prolactinoma or hypothyroidism.
   b. Periodic progestin cycling is necessary to prevent endometrial hyperplasia from unopposed estrogen.
   c. Ovulation induction with clomiphene citrate is necessary if pregnancy is desired.

2. The **PCT is negative** if no bleeding occurs. This results either from inadequate estrogen or an outflow tract obstruction. A combined estrogen–progesterone challenge test (EPCT) clarifies the etiology of amenorrhea.

C. An **EPCT should be administered** (conjugated estrogen 1.25 mg PO for 21 days followed by medroxyprogesterone acetate 10 mg PO for 7 days) to see whether withdrawal bleeding occurs.

1. An **EPCT is positive** if any bleeding beyond a few drops occurs within 2–7 days. This always results from **lack of estrogen.**
   a. An FSH level should be obtained to distinguish between **hypothalamic-pituitary failure** (low FSH) or **ovarian failure** (high FSH). If FSH is low, CNS imaging should be obtained to rule out a tumor.
   b. **Estrogen** should be provided to prevent sequelae of estrogen deficiency, along with **cyclic progestins** to prevent endometrial hyperplasia, regardless of the specific cause.

2. An **EPCT is negative** if no bleeding occurs. This is always due to an **outflow tract obstruction.** Obtain a **hysterosalpingogram (HSG)** to identify the site of the obstruction (e.g., cervical stenosis) and rule out endometrial adhesions (Asherman's syndrome).

Clinical Situation 16–1

Basic Case: An adolescent girl is brought by her mother to the outpatient office. The daughter has never had a menstrual period.

Patient Snapshot	Intervention	Clinical Pearls
She is **13 years of age without** breast development or pubic hair.	Manage conservatively. Developmental findings are within normal range.	**Primary amenorrhea** is diagnosed with age > 14 years and with **absence** of secondary sex characteristics.
She is **15 years of age without** breast development or pubic hair. Pelvic exam shows normal vagina and uterus.	Obtain FSH and karyotype.	_Turners_ **Gonadal dysgenesis** has ↑ FSH and 45,X. **Hypothalamic-pituitary dysfunction** has ↓ FSH and 46,XX.
She is **15 years of age with** breast development and pubic hair. Pelvic exam shows normal vagina and uterus.	Manage conservatively. Clinical findings are within normal range.	**Primary amenorrhea** is diagnosed with age > 16 years and with **presence** of secondary sex characteristics.
She is **17 years of age with** breast development and pubic hair. Pelvic exam shows short vagina and absent uterus.	Obtain serum testosterone and karyotype.	The two primary etiologies to consider are **müllerian agenesis** (normal testosterone; 46,XX) and **androgen insensitivity** (↑ testosterone; 46,XY).
She is **17 years of age with** breast development and pubic hair. Pelvic exam shows normal vagina and uterus.	Perform same workup as for secondary amenorrhea (see Chapter 16 III).	**Estrogen** must be produced by the gonads to stimulate **breast development.**

FSH = follicle-stimulating hormone

βhcg , Pct

Clinical Situation 16–2

Basic Case: A 21-year-old nonpregnant woman states that she has not had a menstrual period for the past few months. A urine β-hCG test is negative.

Patient Snapshot	Intervention	Clinical Pearls
Her menses have been irregular. She displays no signs of virilization.	Perform a PCT.	A **PCT** determines whether the problem is a hormonal deficit (either estrogen or progesterone) or an outflow tract problem.
➡ MPA is given for 7 days, after which she **does** have a withdrawal bleed.	Obtain serum TSH and serum prolactin.	A **positive PCT** results from **anovulation** (adequate estrogen but no progesterone). Rule out correctable causes of anovulation.
➡ **Scenario 1** Serum prolactin is ↑	Obtain sella turcica imaging study.	Excess prolactin from a pituitary **prolactinoma** can inhibit GnRH, resulting in anovulation.
➡ **Scenario 2** Serum TSH and serum prolactin are normal.	Give periodic cycling with progestin.	Progestin cycling prevents unopposed estrogen stimulation that could lead to endometrial hyperplasia.
MPA is given for 7 days, after which she **does not** have a withdrawal bleed.	Perform EPCT.	A **negative PCT** results from either lack of estrogen or obstruction of the outflow tract. The **EPCT** distinguishes between these two etiologies.
CEE is given for 21 days followed by MPA for 7 days. She **does** have a withdrawal bleed.	Obtain serum FSH.	A **positive EPCT** indicates inadequate estrogen. The FSH helps identify the reason for the estrogen deficiency.
➡ FSH is high.	Obtain karyotype to rule out mosaicism.	**Ovarian follicle failure** is the cause of the low estrogen level. At this age, it may be caused by chromosomal mosaicism with a Y chromosome. This has cancer potential.
➡ FSH is low.	Obtain CNS imaging to rule out hypothalamic-pituitary lesion.	**Hypothalamic-pituitary failure** has led to absence of ovarian follicles stimulation, thus the low estrogen level. Imaging studies rule out a CNS lesion.
CEE is given for 21 days followed by MPA for 7 days. She **does not** have a withdrawal bleed.	Obtain an HSG.	A **negative EPCT** indicates the problem is not hormonal deficiency but an **outflow tract obstruction** of Asherman's syndrome.

CEE = conjugated equine estrogen	GnRH = gonadotropin-releasing hormone	MPA = medroxyprogesterone acetate
CNS = central nervous system	hCG = human chorionic gonadotropin	PCT = progesterone challenge test
EPCT = estrogen–progesterone challenge test	HSG = hysterosalpingogram	TSH = thyroid-stimulating hormone

17

Menstrual-Endocrine Abnormalities

I. ABNORMAL MENSTRUAL BLEEDING (Figure 17–1) This condition is diagnosed when any one of the following normal criteria are not met.

A. Criteria for normal ovulatory menstrual cycles

1. **Cycle length:** between 21 and 35 days

2. **Cycle duration:** between 2 and 7 days

3. **Flow volume (per cycle):** < 80 ml

4. **Regularity:** generally predictable from month to month

B. Etiologic classification

1. No identifiable organic causes
a. Cycles are **anovulatory,** with unpredictable, irregular bleeding. This is often referred to as **"dysfunctional uterine bleeding."**
b. Usual causes are **hormonal·deficiencies** or **excesses.**

2. Identifiable structural or anatomic causes
a. Cycles are **ovulatory** and predictable, with bleeding occurring between cycles.
b. Usual causes are **endometrial polyps** or **submucous leiomyomas.**

C. Differential diagnosis

1. **Vaginal conditions:** atrophy, trauma, infection, malignancy

2. **Cervical conditions:** eversion, inflammation, polyps, malignancy

3. **Uterine conditions:** miscarriage, molar pregnancy, endometritis, polyps, submucous myoma, adenomyosis, hyperplasia, malignancy

4. **Tubal conditions:** salpingitis, ectopic pregnancy, malignancy

5. **Ovarian conditions:** estrogen-producing tumors, malignancy

D. Diagnostic workup

1. **Rule out pregnancy** with a qualitative urine or serum β-human chorionic gonadotropin (β-hCG) test. Pregnancy is the *most common* cause of abnormal bleeding in the reproductive years.

2. **Perform endometrial biopsy** in anovulatory patients only when serious endometrial pathology is likely **(Figure 17–2). Biopsy is not necessary** when the likelihood of atypical endometrial hyperplasia is low (e.g., in adolescence when anovulation is common in the first 2 years after menarche).

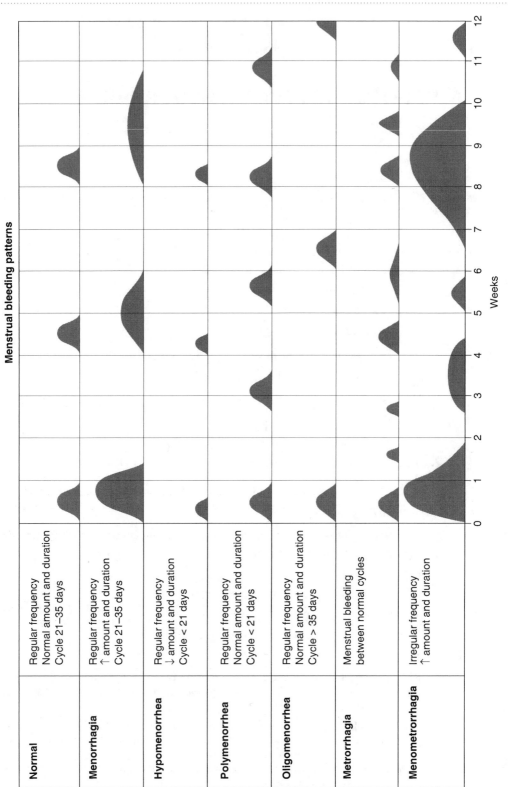

Figure 17–1. Menstrual bleeding. (From Sakala EP: *BRS Obstetrics and Gynecology*, 2nd ed. Philadelphia, Lippincott Williams & Wilkins, 2000, p 304.)

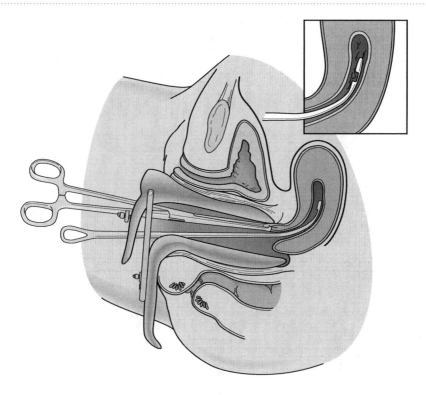

Figure 17–2.   Endometrial biopsy. After a small curette is passed into the endometrial cavity, samples of the endometrium may be obtained by curettage or aspiration.

    a. Biopsy selected patients during their reproductive years, when the risk of endometrial hyperplasia or carcinoma is moderate [e.g., age > 35 years; presence of obesity, hypertension, or diabetes mellitus (DM)].

    b. Biopsy all patients after menopause, when the risk of endometrial hyperplasia or carcinoma is high.

E. Management

    1. If cycles appear anovulatory (Table 17–1):

        a. Initiate a progestin trial [medroxyprogesterone acetate (MPA) 10 mg PO for 10 days]. Expect the following events to occur if cycles are anovulatory:

          (1) Bleeding should stop within 48 hours of starting the trial.

          (2) Bleeding should remain stopped until the trial is completed.

          (3) Normal withdrawal bleeding should occur after the trial is completed.

        b. If the progestin trial confirms anovulation, take the following steps:

          (1) Determine if causes of anovulation are correctable using the following tests:

            (a) Prolactin level, which can rule out pituitary prolactinoma

            (b) Thyroid-stimulating hormone (TSH) level, which can rule out hypothyroidism

          (2) Treat with periodic MPA cycling to prevent endometrial hyperplasia due to unopposed estrogen.

Table 17–1
Comparison of Ovulatory and Anovulatory Cycles

Characteristics	Ovulatory Cycles	Anovulatory Cycles
Predictability	*Predictable*	*Unpredictable*
Hormonal stimulation	Estrogen–progesterone withdrawal	Estrogen stimulation only (unopposed estrogen)
Endometrial stability	**Stable** (no random breakdown)	**Unstable** (frequent random breakdown)
Time and site of menstrual changes	**Simultaneous** (all endometrial segments)	**Random**
Nature of tissue breakdown	*Orderly, progressive*	*Spontaneous, haphazard*
Duration of bleeding	*Self-limited* due to spiral arteriolar constriction	*Prolonged* due to absence of vasoconstriction
Basal body temperature	Midcycle elevation	No elevation
Endometrial biopsy	Secretory changes	Proliferative changes only

2. If cycles appear ovulatory (see Table 17–1):
   a. Look for structural lesions in the endometrium.
   (1) With saline infusion sonography. Instill saline into the uterus with a transcervical catheter, and then visualize the lesions in the uterine cavity by endovaginal sonography.
   (2) With hysteroscopy. Visualize the lesions in the uterine cavity directly with a fiberoptic scope.
   (3) With endometrial curettage. Scrape the endometrial cavity.
   b. Resect any endometrial polyps or submucous myomas using an operating hysteroscope.

3. With a failed progestin trial and no apparent endometrial lesions:
   a. Provide medical treatment with the following agents: nonsteroidal anti-inflammatory drugs (NSAIDs), oral contraceptives, or danazol.
   b. Perform iatrogenic scarring of the endometrium. Reduce bleeding by an endometrial ablation method, using a heating element to produce thermal injury. This may include microwave, laser, rollerball, or balloon methods.
   c. Perform hysterectomy as a last resort if response to medical or conservative surgical management is inadequate.

II. DYSMENORRHEA. This condition is characterized by **excessive pain with menses** so severe that it alters a woman's daily activities.

   A. Primary dysmenorrhea

   1. Definition. Primary dysmenorrhea is excessive menstrual pain and cramping arising at the onset of ovulatory cycles within 2 years of menarche.

   2. Pathophysiology. Uterine pain results from prostaglandin-mediated uterine ischemia caused by progesterone withdrawal.

   3. Diagnosis
   a. A history of menses-related lower abdominal-pelvic cramping associated with **prostaglandin-related symptoms** (nausea, vomiting, diarrhea, headache) is characteristic.
   b. Pelvic examination is normal, without pathology.

4. Management. Goals are either inhibition of prostaglandin production or suppression of progesterone withdrawal. **Therapeutic agents** include prostaglandin synthetase inhibitors, NSAIDs, and oral contraceptives.

B. Secondary dysmenorrhea

1. Definition. Secondary amenorrhea is excessive menstrual pain and cramping arising in the midreproductive years, usually with identifiable anatomic pathology.

2. Pathophysiology. Disease development varies depending on etiology. Causes include **endometriosis, pelvic adhesions,** adenomyosis, leiomyomas, and cervical stenosis.

3. Diagnosis

a. A **history** of menses-related lower abdominal-pelvic pain that is often dull and aching is characteristic. **Associated symptoms** may include infertility, painful intercourse **(dyspareunia),** painful defecation **(dyschezia),** and abnormal vaginal bleeding.

b. Pelvic examination is variable, depending on specific pathology.

c. Diagnostic tests (see Chapter 21 II, III)

(1) Pelvic sonography can detect abnormalities in size or shape of a uterus with leiomyomas or adenomyosis.

(2) Diagnostic laparoscopy is necessary to confirm endometriosis and pelvic adhesions.

4. Management. Treatment varies according to the pathology identified in the clinical workup.

III. ENDOMETRIOSIS. In this condition, the endometrial glands and stroma are found outside the uterine cavity. **Prevalence** is highest in multiparas during the fourth and fifth decade of life.

A. Pathophysiology. The *most common* location of lesions is the **ovary,** followed by the cul-de-sac, uterosacral ligaments, broad ligaments, and oviducts **(Figure 17–3).** These anatomic locations are consistent with a **retrograde menstruation** theory of pathogenesis.

B. Symptoms

1. Primary complaints include dysmenorrhea, dyspareunia, dyschezia, and infertility.

2. Symptom severity may be unrelated to the extent of disease. Extensive disease may be asymptomatic, yet minimal disease may be associated with major morbidity.

C. Clinical findings (variable). Classic signs include a retroverted uterus with uterosacral ligament nodularity and tenderness. Ovarian endometriomas present as adnexal masses.

D. Diagnosis. Laparoscopic visualization of lesions, which vary from small peritoneal bluish implants to dense adhesions involving the entire pelvis, are the basis of diagnosis.

E. Management

1. Medical therapy aims to cause atrophy of endometrial tissue with **pseudopregnancy** (continuous progestins) or **pseudomenopause** (danazol, an antiestrogen; leuprolide, a gonadotropin-releasing hormone [GnRH] agonist).

2. Surgical therapy may be **conservative** (adhesion lysis for fertility treatment) or **radical** (pelvic cleanout [TAH, BSO] for pain relief).

Figure 17–3. Clinical features of endometriosis.

IV. PREMENSTRUAL DISORDERS

A. Overview. Premenstrual disorders encompass a complex combination of "physical" and "emotional" (or behavioral) symptoms that occur premenstrually and are absent for the rest of the cycle; the symptoms are severe enough to significantly interfere with work or home activities. **Symptoms are absent in the first half of the cycle.** The severity of symptoms occurs on a continuum ranging from mild to moderate to severe. Three diagnoses can be used depending on the degree of symptom severity.

1. **Premenstrual symptoms** are recognized in the majority of women in the reproductive years but do not interfere with their normal functioning.

2. **Premenstrual Syndrome (PMS)** is diagnosed when the physical and emotional symptoms interfere with normal functioning. With PMS, sadness or mild depression is not uncommon.

3. **Premenstrual Dysphoric Disorder (PMDD).** The physical symptom list is identical for PMS and PMDD; while the emotional symptoms are similar, they are significantly more serious with PMDD. In PMDD, the criteria focus on the mood rather than the physical symptoms. With PMDD, however, significant depression and hopelessness may occur.

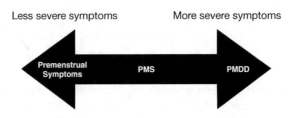

B. Pathogenesis. The etiology of PMS is unclear but is probably **multifactorial.** Suggested theories include estrogen–progesterone imbalance, vitamin deficiencies, serotonin deficiency, and renin–angiotensin imbalance.

C. Clinical findings

   1. Symptom pattern. The specific symptoms are less important than their **recurrent, temporal relationship** to the menstrual cycle. The **first week of the cycle should be symptom-free,** and the symptoms that appear during the second half of the cycle should completely disappear with onset of menses.

   2. Specific symptoms (may be variable)
   a. Emotional symptoms: depression, irritability, mood swings
   b. Fluid retention–associated symptoms: breast tenderness, edema, weight gain, bloating
   c. Musculoskeletal symptoms: muscle aches, joint pain, headache

   3. Clinical examination. No specific physical findings are diagnostic.

   4. Diagnosis. The patient keeps a **menstrual diary** in which she records the nature and intensity of specific symptoms on each day of her menstrual cycle. Conditions that conform to the previously described temporal pattern confirm the diagnosis (see IV C 1).

D. Management. Treatment is based on the predominant symptom cluster.

   1. Selective serotonin reuptake inhibitors (SSRIs) are the only treatment for severe emotional symptoms shown effective in randomized, double blind studies. Intermittent therapy, with the SSRI given only during the symptomatic phase, has been as helpful as continuous therapy. Agents used include fluoxetine (Prozac) 20–60 mg/day, paroxetine (Paxil), and sertaline (Zoloft) 50–150 mg/day.

   2. Spironolactone, a potassium-sparing diuretic, may be helpful for fluid retention symptoms (100 mg/day) during the luteal phase.

   3. NSAIDs may be helpful for musculoskeletal complaints.

   4. Oral contraceptives may help normalize hormonal fluctuations.

   5. Gonadotropin-releasing hormone (GnRH) agonists have improved symptoms but the hypoestrogenic side effects and cost limit usefulness.

   6. Bilateral salpingo-oophorectomy (BSO) is controversial because it is irreversible. It is reserved for most severely affected patients who fail medical therapy.

V. HIRSUTISM

A. Definitions

   1. Hirsutism is excess growth of **male-pattern,** pigmented, terminal hairs on the body midline (e.g. face, upper lip, chin, chest, abdomen, back, inner thighs) **[Figure 17–4].** This condition may be physiologic.

   2. Virilization is excess male-pattern hair as well as increased muscle mass, clitorimegaly, temporal balding, and deepening voice. **This condition is always pathologic.**

   3. Hypertrichosis is excess nonsexual hair (e.g. eyebrows, eyelashes, forearms, lower legs).

B. Pathophysiology

   1. Vellus hair (lightly pigmented, finely textured) converts to **terminal hair** (darkly pigmented and coarse) under the influence of **androgens.**

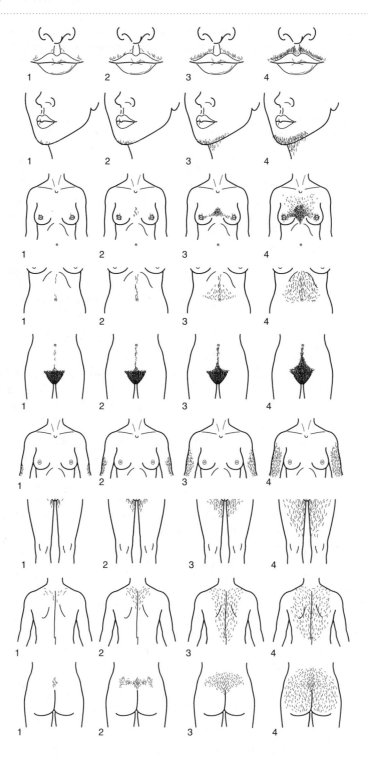

Figure 17–4. Hirsutism in nine body areas, scoring from 1 (mild) to 4 (severe). A total score exceeding 8 indicates hirsutism. (After Scott JR, DiSaia PJ, Hammond CB et al [eds]: *Danforth's Obstetrics and Gynecology*, 6th ed. Philadelphia, JB Lippincott, 1990.)

2. Axillary hair and **pubic hair** have **low thresholds** of androgen sensitivity. Even the relatively low levels of adrenal androgens that occur during puberty are enough to convert axillary and vellus hair to terminal hair in normal females.

3. Face, upper lip, chin, and chest hair have **high threshold** of androgen sensitivity. **In males,** conversion of vellus hair to terminal hair in these sites normally occurs in the presence of high levels of circulating testicular androgens. **In females,** conversion to terminal hair in these sites does not normally take place, but may occur in two ways:

  a. Increased circulating free androgens are produced in abnormal quantities by either the ovaries or adrenal glands.

  b. Increased 5α-reductase enzyme activity in the hair follicle converts testosterone to the highly potent dihydrotestosterone. This etiology is often referred to as "idiopathic" or hair-follicle sensitivity. Free androgens are at normal female levels.

C. Differential diagnosis

  1. Ovarian etiologies of elevated androgens are identified by serum **testosterone** levels.

  a. Polycystic ovarian (PCO) syndrome. In this common disorder of long duration, onset after puberty is gradual. Anovulation, infertility, and obesity are common. Testosterone levels are mildly elevated. A serum luteinizing hormone/follicle-stimulating hormone (LH/FSH) ratio of > 3 suggests PCO syndrome.

  b. Androgen-producing tumor. In this rare disorder of short duration, onset is rapid. Physical examination reveals unilateral pelvic mass and virilization changes (e.g., clitorimegaly). Testosterone levels are markedly elevated. The *most common* tumors are Sertoli-Leydig cell and hilar cell tumors.

  2. Adrenal etiologies of elevated androgens are identified by serum **dehydroepiandrosterone sulfate (DHEAS)** and **17-OH progesterone (17-OHP)** levels, as well as the **dexamethasone suppression test (DST).**

  a. Androgen-producing tumor. Onset is rapid after puberty of short duration. Physical examination reveals virilization changes (e.g., clitorimegaly). Imaging studies show abdominal mass. DHEAS levels are markedly elevated. The *most common* tumors are adenomas.

  b. Late-onset congenital adrenal hyperplasia. This rare autosomal dominant condition is due to a 21-hydroxylase enzyme deficiency. Onset is gradual after puberty. Menstrual irregularities are common, and 17-OHP levels are elevated.

  c. Cushing syndrome. Increased levels of adrenocorticotropic hormone (ACTH) lead to excess adrenal glucocorticoid production. Menstrual irregularities are common. Physical examination shows central obesity, dorsal neck fat pad, and abdominal striae. Diagnosis is confirmed by failure to suppress cortisol with an overnight DST.

  3. Hair follicle androgen sensitivity (idiopathic) is often a diagnosis of exclusion after ovarian and adrenal causes are ruled out by normal levels of testosterone, DHEAS, and 17-OHP. Family history is often positive, and ethnic background is Mediterranean. Onset is gradual after puberty, with long duration.

D. Diagnosis (Table 17–2)

E. Management

  1. Discontinue **exogenous androgenic medications.**

Table 17–2
Diagnostic Workup for Hirsutism

HISTORY

Finding	Possible Etiology
Ethnic or **family history**	Idiopathic (hair follicle androgen sensitivity)
Gradual onset after puberty	PCO, CAH, or idiopathic etiology
Rapid onset any time	Androgenic tumor of ovary or adrenal
Onset during pregnancy	Luteoma or theca lutein cysts
Irregular menses and **infertility**	PCO syndrome

PHYSICAL EXAMINATION

Finding	Possible Etiology
Virilization	Androgenic tumor of ovary or adrenal
Obesity	PCO syndrome or Cushing syndrome
Unilateral adnexal mass	Androgenic ovarian tumor
Bilateral adnexal masses in pregnancy	Luteoma or theca lutein cysts

in pregnancy

LABORATORY TESTING

Finding	Possible Etiology
Serum total **testosterone**	High value suggests ovarian tumor
Serum **DHEAS**	High value suggests adrenal tumor
Serum **17-OHP**	High value suggests CAH
Dexamethasone suppression test	High cortisol value suggests Cushing syndrome
Serum **LH/FSH ratio**	Ratio > 3 suggests PCO syndrome

CAH = congenital adrenal hyperplasia   FSH = follicle-stimulating hormone   17-OHP = 17-OH progesterone
DHEAS = dehydroepiandrosterone sulfate   LH = luteinizing hormone   PCO = polycystic ovarian

2. **With ovarian or adrenal tumors,** surgically remove the neoplasm.

3. **With congenital adrenal hyperplasia,** administer **glucocorticoids** to suppress adrenal overproduction of 17-OHP.

4. **With PCO syndrome,** administer **oral contraceptives** to suppress gonadotropin stimulation of ovarian androgen. Oral contraceptives also raise sex hormone–binding globulin levels, thus lowering free androgen levels.

5. **With idiopathic etiology,** administer **spironolactone** to suppress 5α-reductase enzyme activity in the hair follicle. Finasteride has not been studied in women. If used in early pregnancy, anomalies of external genitalia can occur in male fetuses.

6. Eflornithine (Vaniqa) cream may be used to reduce unwanted facial hair. It shows hair growth by blocking differentiation of cells within hair follicles.

7. **Remove unwanted hair** with cosmetic measures (e.g., electrolysis, shaving, waxing).

Clinical Situation 17–1

Basic Case: A woman comes to the office with a 6-month history of abnormal menstrual bleeding.

Patient Snapshot	Intervention	Clinical Pearls
She is **15 years of age.** Her bleeding is unpredictable and irregular.	Obtain qualitative urine or serum β-hCG.	During the reproductive years, regardless of patient age, the first step is to **rule out pregnancy.**
➥ 1 hour later: The lab reports that the urine β-hCG is negative.	Prescribe progestin cycling to prevent endometrial hyperplasia.	After menarche, it takes 2 years for anovulatory (estrogen-dominant) cycles to convert to ovulatory (estrogen–progesterone withdrawal) cycles. Atypical hyperplasia risk is negligible, so there is no need to perform endometrial biopsy.
She is **30 years of age.** Bleeding is unpredictable and irregular. She weighs 130 lb and is 5′3″ tall. BP is 125/70 mm Hg. Urine β-hCG is negative.	Prescribe progestin cycling. No endometrial biopsy is necessary.	Unpredictable bleeding is most likely **anovulatory** from unopposed estrogen. Progestin stabilizes the endometrium and should lead to regular cycles again.
She is **30 years of age.** Bleeding is unpredictable and irregular. She weighs 180 lb and is 5′3″ tall. BP is 155/90 mm Hg. Urine β-hCG is negative.	Perform endometrial biopsy.	Even though she is young, she has **obesity** and **hypertension,** which are risk factors for endometrial carcinoma. Endometrial biopsy is essential to rule out atypical hyperplasia or carcinoma.
She is **30 years of age.** Bleeding is predictable, occurring between regular cycles. She weighs 135 lb and is 5′4″ tall. BP is 125/70 mm Hg. Urine β-hCG is negative.	Perform hysteroscopy or saline hysterosonography and then D&C.	Abnormal bleeding between regular cycles is unlikely to be due to anovulation. Most likely it results from an **anatomic or structural lesion.** Visualization of the lesion is necessary.
➥ 1 day later: saline hysterosonography shows a 3 × 4-cm endometrial polyp.	Perform hysteroscopic removal of the polyp.	Either a **polyp or submucous leiomyoma** can be surgically resected with an operative hysteroscopy.

BP = blood pressure   D&C = dilation and curettage   hCG = human chorionic gonadotropin

Clinical Situation 17–2

Basic Case: A nulligravida comes to the office with a history of menstrual cramps.

Patient Snapshot	Intervention	Clinical Pearls
She is 17 years of age and has a 2-year history of menstrual cramps so painful that she cannot function. The pain is associated with nausea, vomiting, and diarrhea.	Perform a pelvic exam.	It is important to rule out **inflammatory** or **infectious** etiology of pelvic pain.
➔ A general and pelvic exam shows normal anatomy without pathology.	Manage with reassurance, **NSAIDs,** or oral contraceptives.	The normal pelvic exam suggests **primary dysmenorrhea.** The goal of treatment is suppression of prostaglandins.
She is 25 years of age and has a 3-year history of dull, aching pain with menses. Other symptoms are pain with intercourse and infertility. On pelvic exam, you find a tender, retroverted uterus and uterosacral ligament nodularity.	Perform diagnostic laparoscopy.	The scenario suggests **endometriosis** as the etiology of **secondary dysmenorrhea.** Definitive diagnosis requires visualization of lesions.
➔ 1 week later: Laparoscopy confirms widespread pelvic endometriosis.	Use medical or surgical therapy, depending on fertility planning.	**Pseudopregnancy** or pseudomenopause seeks to enhance lesion atrophy medically. Surgical therapy can be conservative or radical.

NSAID = nonsteroidal anti-inflammatory drug

Clinical Situation 17–3

Basic Case: A 25-year-old multigravida comes to the office for a routine visit.

Patient Snapshot	Intervention	Clinical Pearls
She complains of depression, mood swings, and weight gain prior to her menses.	Have patient keep a **menstrual diary** for 3 months.	The diary helps identify specific symptoms and their relationship to her cycles.
➔ **Scenario 1** (3 months later): Her diary shows that her depression and mood swings are present continuously.	Initiate a workup or refer patient for depression.	True PMS symptoms are not present continuously but occur cyclically.
➔ **Scenario 2** (3 months later): Her diary shows that her depression and mood swings are consistently absent in the first 2 weeks of her cycle but are consistently present in the 2 weeks prior to menses.	Start patient on SSRIs for her symptoms.	SSRIs do not help all PMS symptoms but are effective for those that are primarily emotional.

PMS = premenstrual syndrome   SSRI = selective serotonin reuptake inhibitor

Clinical Situation 17–4

Basic Case: A 25-year-old woman comes to the office with concerns about excessive darkly pigmented hair on her chin, upper lip, abdomen, and thighs.

Patient Snapshot	Intervention	Clinical Pearls
Onset of excessive hair has been rapid over the last 3 months. The woman states that her clitoris has enlarged.	Perform complete exam. Obtain serum testosterone and DHEAS.	**Rapid onset** of symptoms, especially with **virilization**, suggests an androgen-producing ovarian or adrenal tumor.
➡ Pelvic exam reveals a solid right adnexal mass and confirms clitorimegaly. Serum testosterone is markedly elevated.	Perform surgical resection of ovarian tumor.	**Sertoli-Leydig** ovarian tumor is likely with high serum **testosterone.** If the serum **DHEAS** were increased, an adrenal tumor would be suspected.
Onset of excessive hair has been gradual since puberty. Her mother and sister have similar findings. Exam does not show evidence of virilization.	Obtain serum testosterone and 17-OHP.	It is important to rule out late-onset CAH (21-OH deficiency), which results in ↑ **17-OHP** levels. Such increases have androgenic effects.
➡ **Scenario 1** Labs—serum 17-OHP, WNL; **testosterone,** mild **elevation.** She has a history of irregular menses and infertility.	Prescribe oral contraceptive pills.	Oral contraceptives help **PCO syndrome** in two ways: they suppress LH, which stimulates ↑ testosterone production; they also increase SHBG, which reduces free testosterone by ↑ binding of testosterone.
➡ **Scenario 2** Labs—serum **17-OHP, elevated.**	Use glucocorticoid replacement.	When given to patients with **CAH,** physiologic doses of prednisone suppress ACTH, which drives adrenal overproduction of androgenic 17-OHP.
Onset of excessive hair has been gradual since puberty. She does not show any virilization. Testosterone, DHEAS, and 17-OHP are all WNL.	Give spironolactone to suppress hair follicle 5α-reductase enzyme activity.	In **idiopathic hirsutism,** systemic androgen levels are normal. Suppression of 5α-reductase activity reduces conversion of low-potency androgens to high-potency ones.

ACTH = adrenocorticotrophic hormone LH = luteinizing hormone SHBG = sex hormone–binding globulin
CAH = congenital adrenal hyperplasia 17-OHP = 17-OH progesterone WNL = within normal limits
DHEAS = dehydroepiandrosterone sulfate PCO = polycystic ovaries

18

Reproductive Life Extremes

I. PRECOCIOUS PUBERTY

A. Overview

    1. **Diagnosis** is made when onset of puberty occurs before the age of 8 years in girls. **Tanner stages I–V** describe the normal development of breasts and pubic hair **(Table 18–1).**

    2. **Incidence** is five times higher in girls than in boys.

B. Terminology

    1. **Isosexual puberty** occurs in the **direction expected** from body phenotype, is mediated by **estrogens,** and is manifested by breast development and female body contours.

    2. **Heterosexual puberty** occurs in the **direction opposite of expected** from body phenotype, is mediated by **androgens,** and is manifested by evidence of virilization.

    3. **Complete puberty** is characterized by the occurrence of all pubertal changes. The *most common* **initial change** is **thelarche** (breast development at 9–10 years of age), followed by **adrenarche** (pubic and axillary hair at 10–11 years), and then **menarche** (onset of menses at age 12–13 years).

    4. **Incomplete puberty** involves only one change—either thelarche, adrenarche, or menarche. This condition is the result of either transient hormone elevation or unusual end-organ sensitivity. Management is conservative.

C. **Etiologic classification** of complete isosexual precocious puberty

    1. **True or central precocity** is mediated by **gonadotropin stimulation** of estrogen production by the ovarian follicles.

        a. **Idiopathic** (unknown etiology) is the *most common* **diagnosis** and involves unexplained premature activation of a normal hypothalamic-pituitary-ovarian (HPO) axis. This condition occurs mostly in girls **over 5 years of age.**

        b. **Central nervous system (CNS) lesions** (e.g., obstructions, infections, tumors) can stimulate the HPO axis by an unknown mechanism. This condition occurs mostly in girls **under 5 years of age.**

    2. **Pseudo or peripheral precocity** is mediated by ovarian production of estrogen independent of **gonadotropin stimulation.**

        a. **McCune-Albright syndrome** (polyostotic fibrous dysplasia) is associated with **café au lait spots** and autonomous ovarian follicle estrogen production.

        b. **Granulosa cell tumor** or fibrothecoma of the ovary may produce estrogen.

Table 18–1
Tanner Developmental Stages in Adolescent Females

Stage	Breast Development	Pubic Hair Development
I	Elevation of areola only	No pubic hair
II	Elevation of breast as a small mound; enlarged areolar diameter	Sparse, long pigmented terminal hair chiefly along labia majora
III	Further enlargement without separation of breasts and areola	Dark, coarse, curled hair sparsely spread over mons
IV	Secondary mound of areola and papilla above the breast; areola pale and immature	Adult-type hair, abundant but limited to the mons
V	Recession of areola to contour of breast; darkening of areola and development of areolar glands and ducts	Adult-type coverage in quantity and distribution with spreading to inner aspects of thighs

D. Management

1. **Gonadotropin-releasing hormone (GnRH) agonists** are used with idiopathic cases of precocity. These agents bind to hypothalamic receptors, suppressing gonadotropin release. When they are discontinued at an appropriate chronologic or physiologic age, normal hormonal cycling resumes.

2. **Medical or surgical therapy** is directed at CNS lesions.

3. **Aromatase inhibitors** are used with McCune-Albright syndrome.

4. **Surgical excision** is used with estrogen-producing ovarian tumors.

E. Prognosis

1. **Short stature** results from premature estrogen-mediated closure of long bone epiphysis.

2. **Sexual functioning and fertility** remain intact.

II. MENOPAUSE

A. Definitions

1. **Natural menopause** occurs after 40 years of age and relates to the time-related depletion of ovarian follicles **(Figure 18–1).** The mean age at menopause is **51 years (Chart 18–1).**

2. **Perimenopause** is the 3- to-5–year period preceding menopause during which ovarian follicle response becomes increasingly unpredictable. As a result, anovulation with amenorrhea and intermittent menopausal symptoms occur.

3. **Premature menopause** may occur between 30 and 40 years of age. It may be idiopathic or occur after oophorectomy or follicle injury caused by radiation, chemotherapy, or infection.

4. **Ovarian failure** may occur prior to age 30. It may be caused by an autoimmune condition or a mosaic karyotype that includes a Y chromosome.

B. Etiology. The underlying event is **loss of functional ovarian follicles,** resulting in low estrogen levels and elevation of gonadotropins. **All symptoms and signs of menopause, whether short-term or long-term, are related to estrogen deficiency.**

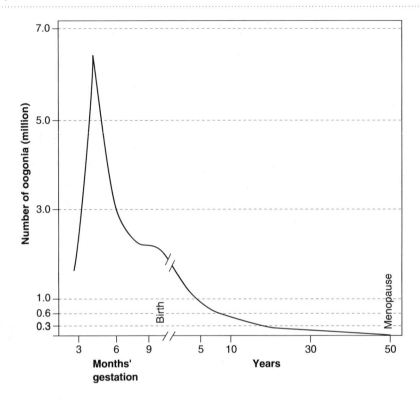

Figure 18–1. Changes in total population of germ cells in the human ovary with increasing age. (Reprinted with permission from Baker TG: *Am J Obstet Gynecol* 110:746, 1971.)

C. Immediate changes

1. Effects on reproductive tract
   a. **Symptoms:** cessation of menses, onset of hot flashes, reversal of premenstrual syndrome (PMS), decreased vaginal lubrication
   b. **Signs:** vaginal epithelial atrophy; decreased size of uterus, cervix, or ovaries; evidence of pelvic diaphragm relaxation such as cystocele, rectocele, or uterine prolapse

2. Effects on urinary tract
   a. **Symptoms:** urinary urgency, frequency, nocturia
   b. **Signs:** urothelial atrophy, urethral caruncle, hypertonic unstable bladder

3. Effects on breasts
   a. **Symptoms:** decreased tenderness
   b. **Signs:** decreased size, fewer benign cysts

4. **Psychological symptoms:** depression, mood swings, irritability

D. Late changes

1. **Osteoporosis** is a disorder of **decreased trabecular bone density** that results from **increased osteoclastic activity.** Bone resorption increases from 0.5% per year before menopause to 5% per year after menopause.
   a. **Risk factors** include positive family history; being **fair-skinned, slender,** and **white;** caffeine intake; smoking; alcohol use; high-protein diet; and inadequate calcium and vitamin D intake.

Life Expectancy and
Age of Menopause

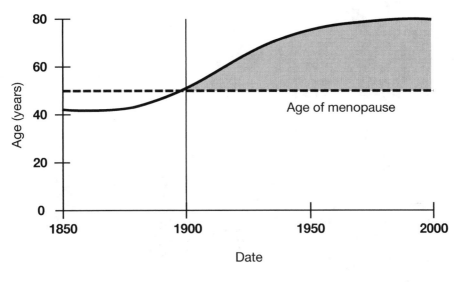

Chart 18–1.

b. Symptoms are **nonexistent** until bone density falls below the fracture threshold. (Vertebral crush fractures are asymptomatic.)

c. Signs include pathologic fractures. The *most common* **fracture site** is the **vertebral body,** resulting in losses of height of up to 3 inches. The next most common fracture sites are the **hip** and **wrist (Chart 18–2).**

d. Diagnosis
   (1) **Current bone density** is measured with **dual energy x-ray absorptiometry (DXA)** scanning.
   (2) **Rate of bone loss** is measured with a **24-hour urine hydroxyproline** assay.

e. Prevention
   (1) **Lifestyle changes** include increased dietary **calcium** and **vitamin D, weight-bearing exercise,** and elimination of cigarettes and alcohol.
   (2) **Medications**
      (a) **Alendronate** (Fosamax), a bisphosphonate medication
      (b) **Raloxifene** (Evista), a **selective estrogen receptor modulator (SERM),** which is an estrogen agonist in bone but an estrogen antagonist in breast and endometrial tissue

2. Cardiovascular disease is the *most common* **cause** of death in women. After menopause the rate of cardiovascular disease in women increases steadily, reaching parity with men by age 70.

a. Lipid profile changes: ↑ in total and LDL cholesterol; ↓ in HDL cholesterol.

b. Prevention includes lifestyle changes (achieving ideal body weight, regular exercise, low fat and low cholesterol diet, avoiding smoking) as well as use of statins (drugs that lower cholesterol by decreasing LDL cholesterol production). Examples of these drugs are lovastatin (Mevacor), pravastatin (Pravachol), and simvastatin (Zocor).

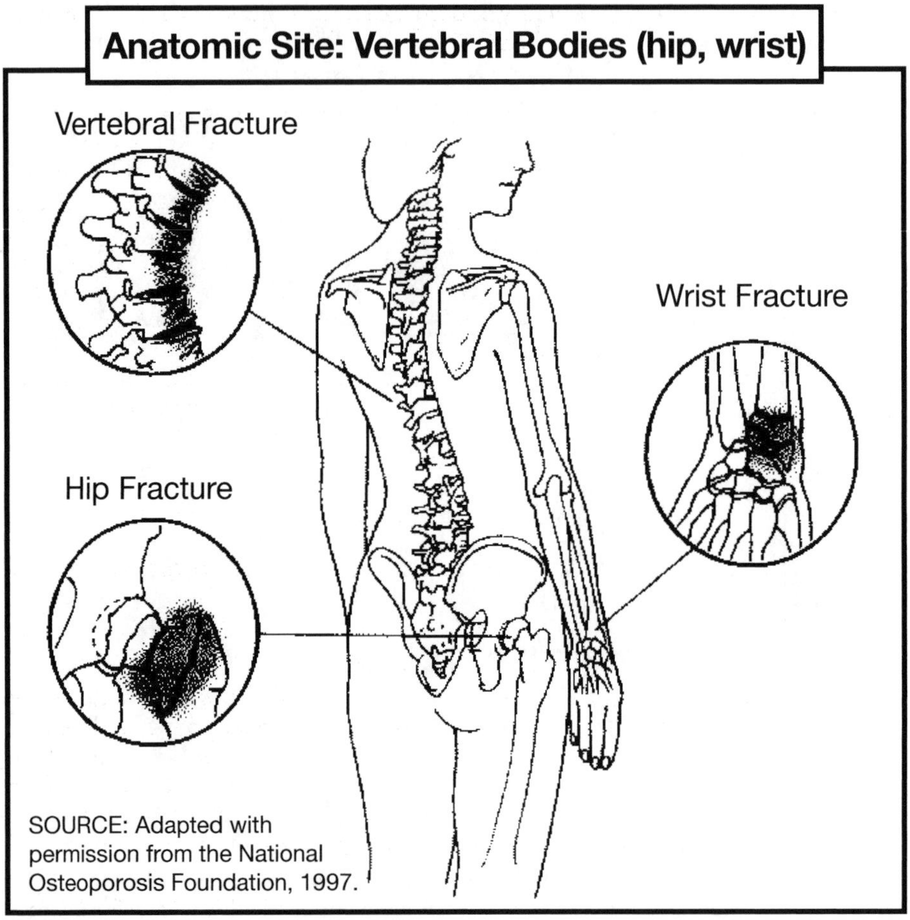

Anatomic Site: Vertebral Bodies (hip, wrist)

Vertebral Fracture

Wrist Fracture

Hip Fracture

SOURCE: Adapted with permission from the National Osteoporosis Foundation, 1997.

Chart 18–2.

E. **Hormone therapy (HT)** may include only estrogen therapy (ET) or combined estrogen plus progestin therapy (EPT).

1. **Benefits**

    a. **Vasomotor symptoms** (hot flushes, night sweats, sleep disturbances) are most pronounced after surgical menopause. They are decreased 80% by HT. **This is the main indication for HT.** Benefits are most dramatic during the first year of treatment.

    b. **Urogenital atrophy** (vaginal dryness, painful intercourse) is significantly improved by HT. **This is another primary indication for HT.** Vaginal administration achieves better symptomatic relief than oral, transdermal, or parental routes.

    c. **Osteoporotic fractures** (hip, vertebral, radius) are decreased by a third with HT. However, because the effect is small, HT should not be used solely for the prevention of fractures.

    d. **Senile dementia** (Alzheimer disease) may be decreased by 40% with HT. This benefit may be dependent on starting HT immediately after menopause. More studies are in process. This is not an indication for HT.

    e. **Endometrial carcinoma** is decreased 10% with HT. This is not an indication for HT.

    f. Colon carcinoma may be decreased by up to 40% with HT. More studies are in process. This is not an indication for HT.

2. **Risks**

    a. Coronary heart disease (CHD) includes nonfatal myocardial infarction and CHD death. While epidemiologic studies show a 40% overall reduction in CHD, randomized controlled trials (RCTs) show a mildly increased risk of HT in women with established CHD. No RCTs have studied the cardioprotective impact of HT in early post-menopausal women without current CHD.

    b. Stroke (mostly ischemic stroke) is mildly increased up to 25% with HT.

    c. Venous thromboembolism (VTE) is a rare complication that includes pulmonary embolus and deep venous thrombosis. Both are increased with HT, with the major increase in the first year and risk declining with continuing use.

    d. Breast cancer is the most common cancer in women. A mildly increased risk of 25% is seen only after five years of EPT. This is comparable with the effect of delayed menopause. Within 5 years after discontinuing EPT, the risk disappears. Risk is not increased with ET.

    e. Ovarian cancer risk increase with HT is controversial.

    f. Gallbladder disease may be increased 2- to 3-fold with HT.

3. **Contraindications** include undiagnosed vaginal bleeding, acute or chronic liver disease, acute vascular thrombosis, hormonally dependent carcinoma (e.g., endometrium, breast).

4. **Administration**

    a. Women with a uterus should be given both estrogen as well as progestin (to prevent endometrial hyperplasia from unopposed estrogen). The route of delivery can be oral, transvaginal, transdermal or injectable. Cyclic estrogen followed by progestin results in predictable withdrawal bleeding. Continuous estrogen and progestin leads to amenorrhea in a few months in most cases.

    b. Women without a uterus should be given estrogen therapy only.

    c. General guidelines

        (1) Vasomotor symptoms and urogenital atrophy are the only indications for HT.

        (2) Lowest dose of HT to relieve symptoms should be used with annual reevaluation.

        (3) Shortest duration of HT should be used with annual re-evaluation. Total duration should not exceed four years.

Clinical Situation 18–1

Basic Case: A 6-year-old girl is brought to the office by her concerned mother, who states that she has seen pubertal changes in her daughter.

Patient Snapshot	Intervention	Clinical Pearls
The girl has not had any bleeding. On exam, pubic hair but no breast development is evident.	Use conservative management.	**Incomplete precocity** is caused by transient hormone elevations or unusual end-organ sensitivity. No treatment is required.
The girl shows female body contours, breast development, and pubic hair.	Obtain a pelvic sonogram to rule out a pelvic mass and an FSH level to assess HPO function.	This is **complete isosexual precocity,** sexual development in the expected female direction. Ovarian estrogens can be mediated by stimulation of the HPO axis (true precocity) or through autonomous production (pseudo precocity).
⇒ **Scenario 1** Pelvic sonogram shows a solid, left adnexal mass. FSH levels are low.	Remove estrogen-producing ovarian tumor.	**Granulosa cell** ovarian tumors can autonomously secrete estrogen independent of GnRH and FSH stimulation from the HPO axis.
⇒ **Scenario 2** Pelvic sonogram is negative. On exam, café au lait skin spots are apparent. FSH levels are low.	Give **testolactone,** an aromatase enzyme inhibitor.	In **McCune-Albright syndrome,** ovarian follicles secrete estrogen independent of GnRH and FSH stimulation
⇒ **Scenario 3** Pelvic sonogram is negative. She complains of headaches and visual changes. FSH levels are elevated.	Order CNS imaging to and rule out tumor, obstruction, or infection	**CNS lesions** can stimulate inappropriate GnRH secretion, resulting in premature activation of normal HPO axis mechanisms. Prognosis is poor.
⇒ **Scenario 4** No adnexal masses are noted. FSH levels are elevated.	Give GnRH agonists to bind to receptors and prevent stimulation.	**Idiopathic etiology** assumes premature activation of normal HPO axis mechanisms. Suppression of GnRH halts the precocity until an appropriate bone age is reached.
The girl shows virilization changes—an enlarged clitoris and facial hair. She has not had any bleeding.	Obtain a pelvic sonogram and abdominal CT scan.	**Heterosexual precocity,** sexual development opposite from expected, is caused in females by increased androgens of ovarian or adrenal origin.
⇒ Pelvic sonogram shows a solid, left adnexal mass.	Remove androgen-producing ovarian tumor.	**Sertoli-Leydig cell** ovarian tumors can autonomously secrete androgens independent of the HPO axis.
⇒ Pelvic sonogram and CT scan are negative.	Rule out CAH.	In **CAH,** adrenal enzyme deficiencies result in overproduction of androgenic precursors.

CAH = congenital adrenal hyperplasia
CNS = central nervous system
CT = computed tomography
FSH = follicle-stimulating hormone
GnRH = gonadotropin releasing hormone
HPO = hypothalamic-pituitary-ovarian

19

Fertility Regulation

I. CONTRACEPTION

A. Effectiveness. For a given contraceptive method, higher effectiveness means a lower failure rate.

    1. Theoretical effectiveness refers to the efficacy of a method when consistent and reliable use—conditions of perfect use—occur.

    2. Actual effectiveness refers to the efficacy when forgetfulness and improper use—conditions of typical use—occur.

B. Unreliable contraceptive methods

    1. Coitus interruptus relies on withdrawal of the penis prior to ejaculation. A high degree of discipline is necessary, and semen can escape into the cervical mucus prior to ejaculation.

    2. Postcoital douching involves flushing semen out of the vagina. However, sperm can enter the cervical mucus within 90 seconds of ejaculation.

    3. Prolongation of lactation assumes existence of ovulatory suppression. Although anovulation does occur, the delay in ovulation is variable; it lasts for no more than 3–6 months.

C. Natural family planning. If intercourse on the fertile days of the menstrual cycle is avoided, pregnancy can be prevented.

    1. The key element is identifying the **time of ovulation** and avoiding intercourse 48 hours before and after this time. Ovulation may be predicted based on past menstrual cycles. A **rise in basal body temperature** or a **change in cervical mucus** from watery to sticky may indicate ovulation.

    2. High failure rates (25%) often occur because of insufficient discipline and inability to predict ovulation accurately. Advantages include wide religious and cultural acceptance and lack of exposure to hormones or chemicals.

D. Barrier contraceptives. These methods work by preventing sperm from entering the female upper reproductive tract.

    1. Types available in the United States
        a. Male condom. This sheath is placed on the erect penis prior to insertion into the vagina and ejaculation. Penile sensitivity may be reduced.
        b. Female condom. This blind pouch with two flexible rings is placed in the vagina, with the open end resting outside the vagina. One size fits all. It can be bulky.

    c. Vaginal diaphragm. This latex dome, which is individually fitted, is placed between the posterior vaginal fornix and pubic symphysis that holds spermicidal jelly against the cervix. It can be inserted 1–2 hours before intercourse. Bladder irritation is a side effect.

    d. Cervical cap. This small, cup-like diaphragm is individually fitted so that it can be placed on the cervix up to 2 days before intercourse. The possibility of its becoming dislodged is a concern.

    e. Spermicidal preparations. These include foams, vaginal suppositories, and jellies, which are placed in the vagina. The spermicidal agent **nonoxynol-9,** which attacks the lipid membrane of the sperm head, may also cause irritation of the genital membranes.

2. Advantages include lack of systemic side effects, relatively low cost, and protection against some sexually transmitted diseases (STDs).

3. Disadvantages, which vary according to the specific method, include loss of sexual spontaneity and a relatively high failure rate (due to forgetfulness and improper use) [up to 20%].

E. Intrauterine contraceptive devices (IUDs)

    1. Types available in the United States (Chart 19–1)

      a. Levonorgestrel IUD (Mirena). Replacement is necessary every 5 years, and it may decrease menstrual cramping and bleeding.

      b. Copper-banded IUD (ParaGuard). Replacement is necessary every 7 years, but it may increase menstrual cramping and bleeding.

    2. Mechanisms of action

      a. Altered implantation due to disruption from endometrial maturation

      b. Altered ovum transport due to changed tubal ciliary action

Only IUDs Available
In the United States   Today

COPPER IUS (*ParaGard®*)   **LNG IUS** (*Mirena®*)

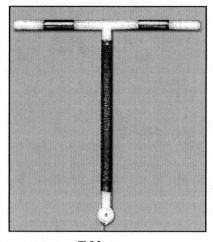
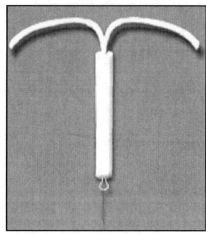

7 Years   **5 Years**

Chart 19–1.

    c. Altered sperm transport from cervix to oviduct

    d. Thickened cervical mucus from progestin effect

    e. Endometrial inflammatory response due to a leukocyte–foreign body reaction

  3. **Contraindications**

    a. **Absolute:** pregnancy; undiagnosed uterine bleeding; acute cervical, uterine, or tubal infection; history of salpingitis; suspected gynecologic malignancy

    b. **Relative:** nulliparity, previous ectopic pregnancy, history of multiple sexual partners or STDs, dysmenorrhea, abnormal uterine cavity, heavy menses, iron deficiency anemia

  4. **Advantages**

    a. High level of effectiveness: failure rate < 2%

    b. Lack of associated systemic metabolic effects

    c. Need for only a single act of motivation for long-term use

  5. **Potential complications**

    a. **Uterine perforation:** rare, with occurrence most likely at the time of insertion, particularly if the uterus is retroverted

    b. **Salpingitis risk:** possibly increased in the first month after placement if STDs are present in the genital tract

    c. ***Actinomyces israeli* colonization of the uterus:** possibly increased

    d. **Septic abortion risk:** 50% with pregnancy occurrence and no IUD removal. (If pregnancy occurs with the IUD in place, the device should be removed immediately.)

F. **Steroid hormone contraception (Table 19–1)**

  1. **Formulations** available in the United States

    a. **Estrogen and progestin pills** are the ***most common* reversible contraceptive** in the United States. These pills are administered orally for 3 weeks with 1 week off to allow for predictable withdrawal bleeding. Failure rate is 2%.

Table 19–1
Comparison of Three Common Steroid Contraceptives

Characteristic	Oral Agent	Injectable Agent	Subcutaneous Agent
Hormone(s)	Estrogen–progestin or progestin only	Progestin only	Progestin only
Pharmacologic name	ESTROGEN PROGESTINS	Depomedroxy- progesterone acetate (DEPO-PROVERA)	l-Norgestrol (NOR-PLANT) [6 Silastic capsules]
Ease of initiation	Easy: self-administered	Easy: by health professional	Complex: by trained health professional
Failure rate	2%–3%	< 1%	< 1%
Mechanism of action	1. Gonadotropin suppression → No ovulation 2. Alteration of cervical mucus → Hostile to sperm 3. Atrophy of endometrium → Unfavorable implantation		
Type of bleeding	Estrogen–progestin: regular, predictable Progestin only: Irregular	Irregular	Irregular
Ease of stopping	No problem	No problem	May be difficult because of scarring
Return of fertility	Prompt	May be delayed up to 18 months	Prompt

(1) **Monophasic types:** fixed amounts of both estrogen and progestin

(2) **Multiphasic types:** a fixed amount of estrogen but a progestin amount that increases incrementally (from week 1 to week 3)

b. **Estrogen and progestin patch** (OrthoEvra) contains ethinyl estradiol (E) and norelgestromin (P) in a transdermal system applied to the upper arm or buttocks. The patches are changed weekly for three weeks followed by a week off to allow for a predictable withdrawal bleed. Failure rate is < 1%, but increases with weight over 200 lb.

c. **Estrogen and progestin vaginal ring** (NuvaRing) contains ethinyl estradiol (E) and etonorgestrel (P) in a transvaginal vinyl ring placed in the vaginal fornices for three weeks after which it is removed to allow for a predictable withdrawal bleed. Failure rate is < 1%.

d. **Progestin-only pills** ("mini-pills"), which are indicated primarily for lactating women, are administered orally continuously but frequently result in breakthrough bleeding (BTB). They are taken every day (without a week off) at the same time each day. Failure rate is 3%.

e. **Progestin-only intramuscular injection** involves the slow release of depomedroxyprogesterone acetate (Depo-Provera). The injection must be repeated **every 3 months.** Failure rate is low (0.3%). Return of ovulation may be delayed up to 18 months, and BTB is common.

f. **Progestin-only subcutaneous depot** involves the placement of silastic progestin-containing capsules under the upper arm skin. **Jadelle** utilizes two levonorgestrel rods, which must be replaced every **5 years. Implanon** utilizes one etonorgestrel rod, which must be replaced every **3 years. Norplant** (with six levonorgestrel rods) is off the market. Failure rates are low (0.2%), but BTB is common. Return of ovulation is prompt after removal of capsules, but removal can be difficult due to scar tissue formation. BTB is common.

2. Mechanisms of action

a. **Gonadotropin suppression,** resulting in anovulation (both estrogen and progestin)

b. **Alteration of cervical mucus,** making it hostile to sperm (progestin only)

c. **Endometrial atrophy,** making it unfavorable to implantation (progestin only)

3. **Contraindications.** These are conditions under which use of steroid contraception may be inadvisable. **Absolute contraindications** mean use is never acceptable. **Relative contraindications** mean use may be acceptable if benefits outweigh risks **(Table 19–2).**

4. **Noncontraceptive health benefits.** Advantages, which include reductions in several pathologic conditions, are largely related to either suppression of ovulation or decreased menstrual flow **(Table 19–3).**

II. STERILIZATION

A. **Methods.** The most commonly used procedures, which are surgical in nature, are designed to occlude the female oviduct or male vas deferens permanently.

1. **Tubal sterilization** is the *most common* **form of pregnancy prevention** used in the United States.

a. This procedure can be performed in the operating room either as an interval procedure or immediately postpartum. Minilaparotomy or laparoscopy is used to ligate or cauterize the oviduct **(Figure 19–1).**

b. No objective criteria for success exist. The **failure rate is 0.5%.** Success in reversing the procedure is variable, with rates as low as 50%.

Table 19–2
Contraindications to Use of Estrogen-Containing Contraceptives

Absolute	Relative
Cardiovascular disease	**Systemic disease**
Venous thrombosis	Diabetes mellitus
Pulmonary embolism	Sickle cell disease
Cerebrovascular accident	Chronic hypertension
Coronary heart disease	Hyperlipidemia
Malignancy	**Neurologic disease**
Breast	Vascular headache
Endometrium	Depression
Melanoma	
Hepatic disease	**Smoking, > 35 years of age**
Liver tumor	
Abnormal liver function tests	
Pregnancy	

   2. Vasectomy is an outpatient procedure performed under local anesthesia. **Objective criteria of success is azoospermia** on a semen collection after twelve ejaculations. The **failure rate is 0.2%.**

B. Regret after sterilization. This reaction is more likely if any of the following criteria are present: age < 30 years, medically indicated procedure, recent emotional trauma, and coercion from spouse or family.

III. INFERTILITY

   A. Definitions

   1. Infertility is the inability of a couple to conceive within 12 months of unprotected intercourse. Prevalence is 10%.

   2. Fecundability is the likelihood of conception occurring in a population of couples within a month. The rate decreases with advancing age of the female partner (20% at age 20, 15% at age 30, 5% at age 40).

Table 19–3
Noncontraceptive Health Benefits of Steroid Contraceptive Agents

Organ	Pathologic Condition *Decreased*
Ovary	Functional ovarian cysts
	Epithelial ovarian cancer
Uterus	Primary and secondary dysmenorrhea
	Dysfunctional uterine bleeding
	Endometrial carcinoma
Oviduct	Pelvic inflammatory disease
	Ectopic pregnancy
Breast	Benign breast disease
Blood	Microcytic iron deficiency anemia
Other	Endometriosis

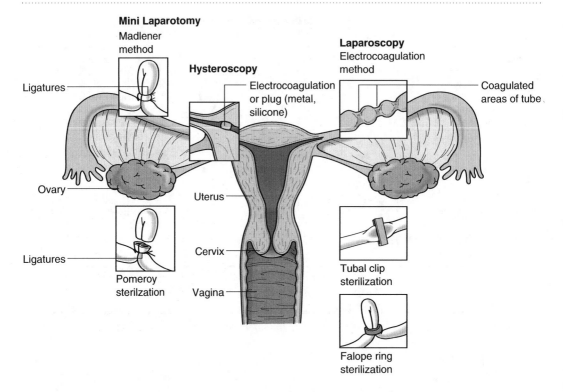

Figure 19–1. Methods of tubal sterilization. (After Clarke-Pearson DL, Dawood MY: *Green's Gynecology: Essentials of Clinical Practice*, 4th ed. Boston, Little, Brown, 1990, p 450.)

B. Etiology (Chart 19–2)

1. **Anovulation** is the *most common* **female cause** of infertility.

    a. **Etiology: polycystic ovarian (PCO) syndrome,** elevated prolactin levels, hypothalamic-pituitary dysfunction, hypothyroidism

    b. **Diagnosis:** history of **unpredictable, irregular menstrual cycles,** absence of midcycle temperature elevation, "midluteal" progesterone level < 3 ng/ml, absence of secretory changes of "midluteal" endometrial biopsy

    c. **Management**

        (1) **Bromocriptine** is used to treat hyperprolactinemia.

        (2) **Clomiphene citrate,** a weak synthetic estrogen that enhances gonadotropin-releasing hormone (GnRH) release, is used as a primary agent for ovulation induction. Hyperstimulation may occur, with a 10% multiple pregnancy rate.

        (3) **Human menopausal gonadotropin,** combined with midcycle human chorionic gonadotropin (hCG), is used with clomiphene failures to trigger ovulation. Hyperstimulation may occur, with a 30% multiple pregnancy rate.

2. **Fallopian tube disease** is the second most common female cause of infertility.

    a. **Etiology:** adhesions from previous pelvic inflammatory disease (PID), ruptured appendix, peritonitis, endometriosis, ectopic pregnancy

    b. **Diagnosis**

        (1) **Hysterosalpingogram (HSG)** identifies intratubal occlusion by failure of peritoneal spillage of radio-opaque media injected into the cervix.

Main Causes of Infertility

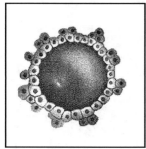

Is there an egg?

A woman's eggs need to be released regularly.

Hormone therapy may help an ovulation problem.

Anovulation

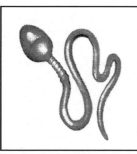

Are there enough sperm?

A man must produce enough active sperm. Hormone therapy or surgery can treat some sperm problems.

Male Factor

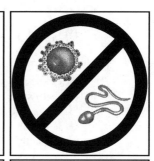

Can egg and sperm meet?

The egg and sperm must be able to meet. Surgery can often treat a blockage in either partner.

Tubal Disease

Chart 19–2.

     (2) **Laparoscopy** identifies external tubal adhesions or disease.
   c. **Management.** Surgically correctable tubal disease is performed laparoscopically using lysis of adhesions or fimbrioplasty.

  3. **Abnormal semen analysis** is the *most common* **male cause** of infertility.
    a. **Etiology:** increased scrotal temperature, smoking, excessive alcohol ingestion, epididymitis, toxins, endocrine disorders
    b. **Diagnosis:** semen analysis performed within 1 hour of ejaculation after 2–7 days of abstinence (normal values: volume 2–5 ml; sperm concentration > 20 million/ml; sperm motility > 50%; normal forms > 70%; pH 7.2–7.8)
    c. **Management**
      (1) **Intrauterine insemination (IUI)** is used with oligozoospermia, mild-to-moderate semen abnormalities, and unexplained infertility.
      (2) **Intracytoplasmic sperm injection (ICSI)** is used with severe semen abnormalities.
      (3) **Donor insemination** is used with azoospermia or failed ICSI.

C. Clinical approach

  1. **Phase I. Inexpensive, noninvasive tests** should be performed first.
    a. **Ovulation** should be documented (see III B 1 b). If cycles are irregular, begin clomiphene for ovulation induction, even though occasional ovulatory cycles may occur.
    b. **Semen analysis** should be repeated in 1 month if it is abnormal (see III B 3 b), because semen quality may vary over time. At least 75% of fertile men have at least one abnormal semen characteristic. If semen analysis is persistently abnormal, IUI and ICSI may be necessary.

    c. **Ovarian reserve** is determined if the female partner is over 35 years of age by obtaining an FSH level on day 3 of her cycle. An elevated FSH level ($>$ 12 mIU/ml) indicates impending ovarian failure.

  2. **Phase II. More expensive, invasive, and painful tests** are performed if ovulation is confirmed and semen analysis is normal.

    a. **HSG** is performed in the proliferative phase just after the menses. If the HSG is normal, ovarian hyperstimulation and IUI can be carried out.

    b. **Diagnostic laparoscopy** is also performed in the proliferative phase only if the HSG shows tubal disease. Tubal repair can be completed at time of surgery if adhesions are found.

    c. **"Unexplained infertility"** is diagnosed if ovulation is occurring, semen analysis is normal, ovarian reserve is confirmed, and no tubal disease is found. Options include **expectant management** or **in vitro fertilization (IVF).**

  3. **Phase III. IVF** is used with severe tubal disease, severe endometriosis, ICSI, or unexplained infertility. Follicle stimulation is followed by ultrasound-guided transvaginal follicle aspiration. Embryos are transferred into the uterus on day 3.

IV. INDUCED ABORTION Abortion is planned pregnancy termination in a manner to ensure nonsurvival of the embryo or fetus

  A. **Risks,** which tend to be higher with advancing gestational age, use of general anesthesia, and maternal systemic diseases, are:

    1. **Uterine perforation** may occur with dilation and curettage (D&C) or dilation and evacuation (D&E).

    2. **Cervical trauma** is more common with second-trimester procedures.

    3. **Bleeding and hemorrhage** occur from the placental site and increase with advancing gestational age.

    4. **Infections** such as endometritis from polymicrobial genital flora tend to occur more often with advancing gestational age.

    5. **Aspiration pneumonitis** may occur when general anesthesia is used.

  B. **First-trimester abortion methods ($<$ 12 weeks).** These procedures tend to be elective.

    1. **Suction D&C,** the *most common* **abortion method** used in the United States, is an outpatient **surgical** procedure performed under local anesthesia or sedation.

      a. After the cervix is dilated, the embryo and placental tissue are aspirated through a cannula with strong vacuum pressure.

      b. Maternal complications are rare, and the maternal mortality rate is 1/100,000.

    2. **Mefipristone (RU-486)** is an oral **progesterone antagonist** used in combination with a prostaglandin to terminate pregnancies **medically** prior to 10 weeks' gestation. Success rates approach 95%, with failures requiring suction D&C.

    3. **Methotrexate,** a **folate antimetabolite** that destroys rapidly growing tissues, is currently seldom used.

  C. **Second-trimester abortion methods (12–24 weeks).** These **surgical** procedures tend to be performed because of fetal anomalies.

    1. **D&E,** which is similar to D&C, is an outpatient procedure. However, cervical dilation must be greater, and fetal tissues can no longer simply be aspirated but must be extracted with surgical instruments. Complications are uncommon. It is the safest second-trimester procedure, with a maternal mortality rate of 4/100,000.

2. Induction of labor is an inpatient procedure with induction-to-delivery intervals of up to 24 hours. General complications can include retained placenta or failed induction. Maternal mortality rate is 8/100,000 (similar to that with term vaginal delivery). Uterine contractions (UCs) may be initiated by one of the following methods:

    a. Intra-amniotic fluid injection of hypertonic saline, hyperosmolar urea, or prostaglandin $F_{2\alpha}$ may result in specific complications such as hypernatremia or disseminated intravascular coagulation (DIC) [hypertonic saline], live birth, nausea, vomiting, and fever (prostaglandins).

    b. Intravaginal placement of prostaglandin E_2 or misoprostol (Cytotec), a prostaglandin E_1 analog, into the vagina may lead to specific complications such as live birth, nausea, vomiting, and fever.

D. Any–gestational age methods. Laparotomy procedures are performed under general anesthesia with maternal mortality rates of **25/100,000,** the highest of any abortion method. They should not be used as primary abortion methods because of their high morbidity and mortality.

    1. Hysterotomy is a mini-cesarean section that is performed only for a failed midtrimester procedure or its complications.

    2. Hysterectomy involves removal of the pregnant uterus because of uncontrolled hemorrhage or invasive cervical cancer prior to viability.

20

Disorders of Pelvic Support

I. PELVIC RELAXATION. This general term refers to the **loss of anatomic support** of the pelvic diaphragm and/or vagina.

 A. Predisposing conditions. Risk factors include aging, estrogen deficiency, pregnancy-associated trauma, genetic predisposition, and chronically increased intra-abdominal pressure.

 B. Terminology

   1. Uterine prolapse. Classification is based on the location of the **cervix.**
      a. First-degree. The cervix is still in the vagina.
      b. Second-degree. The cervix is at the introitus.
      c. Third-degree (procidentia). The uterus and cervix are both prolapsed out of the introitus.

   2. Cystocele (Figure 20–1). The anterior vaginal wall is prolapsed, containing the **bladder.** Symptoms may include urinary urgency, frequency, or incontinence.

   3. Enterocele (see Figure 20–1). The upper posterior vaginal wall is prolapsed, containing the **small bowel.** Symptoms are nonspecific.

   4. Rectocele (see Figure 20–1). The lower posterior vaginal wall is prolapsed, containing the **rectum.** Symptoms include difficulty emptying the rectum, requiring digital pressure in the vagina (digital splinting).

 C. Symptoms. Disorders are primarily asymptomatic, and even when symptoms occur, they are often nonspecific, including backache, pelvic pressure, and difficulty walking.

 D. Examination. With **mild prolapse,** the structures involved are contained within the vagina and are detectable only with the patient straining. With **more advanced prolapse,** the structures are apparent at or beyond the introitus without straining.

 E. Management

   1. Medical approaches
      a. Kegel exercises, which involve voluntary contraction of the pelvic muscles to strengthen tone, may be helpful in cases of mild relaxation.
      b. Estrogen replacement therapy (ERT) can reverse atrophic changes and improve tissue turgor in postmenopausal women.
      c. Pessaries, which are mechanical devices placed in the vagina, place the pelvic structures in a more normal position artificially. This therapy is a temporary treatment for nonsurgical candidates.
      d. Pelvic floor electrical stimulation can improve pelvic floor muscle strength.

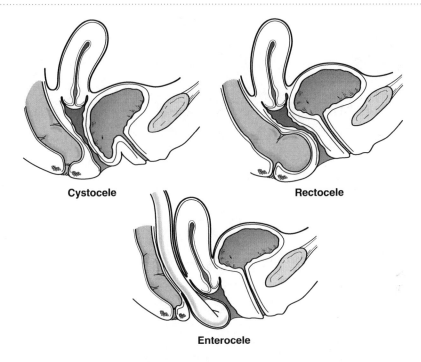

Cystocele   Rectocele

Enterocele

Figure 20–1.   Three types of vaginal prolapse. [Redrawn with permission from Hacker NF, Moore JG (eds): *Essentials of Obstetrics and Gynecology*, 2nd ed. Philadelphia, W.B. Saunders, 1992, p 397.]

    2. Surgical approaches. Definitive treatment involves surgery. The extensiveness of the procedure used depends on the degree of relaxation and patient age.
        a. Anterior and posterior colporrhaphy, which plicates the submucosal fascia in vaginal wall prolapse, is recommended for patients with cystocele or rectocele.
        b. Total hysterectomy, either vaginal or abdominal, is often recommended for uterine prolapse if childbearing is completed.

II. URINARY INCONTINENCE

  A. Physiology of micturition (Chart 20–1)

    1. Continence occurs when urine remains in the bladder. When the bladder is full, voluntary suppression of detrusor contractions normally allows control of involuntary micturition.
        a. Urine remains in the bladder as long as the pressure within the bladder remains less than the pressure within the bladder neck and urethra.
        b. Continence is under control of the **sympathetic nervous system** and is maintained by:
            (1) Detrusor relaxation, which is under **β-adrenergic stimulation**
            (2) Bladder neck contraction, which is under **α-adrenergic stimulation**

    2. Incontinence occurs when urine is lost from the bladder.
        a. Loss of urine takes place when the pressure within the bladder rises above the pressure within the bladder neck and urethra.
        b. Incontinence is under control of the **parasympathetic nervous system** and results from:

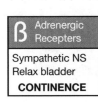

β **Adrenergic Recepters**

Sympathetic NS
Relax bladder
CONTINENCE

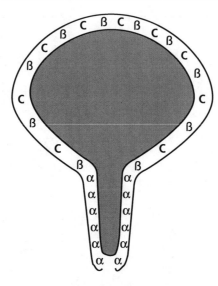

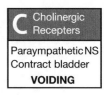

C **Cholinergic Receptors**

Paraympathetic NS
Contract bladder
VOIDING

α **Adrenergic Recepters**

Sympathetic NS
Contract urethra
CONTINENCE

Chart 20–1.

(1) Detrusor muscle contraction, which is under **cholinergic stimulation**
(2) Bladder neck relaxation, which is also under **cholinergic stimulation**

B. **Clinical approach. Evaluate the patient sequentially for the three most common types of incontinence** (stress, hypertonic, and hypotonic) and provide the appropriate treatment (see II C 1–3).

1. **Obtain a urinalysis (UA)—the first, most cost-effective step.** Involuntary detrusor contractions can be caused by bladder irritation due to any of the following pathologic conditions:

a. **Cystitis.** UA is positive for **bacteria and leukocytes.** Cystitis is treated on an outpatient basis with a single oral antibiotic.

b. **Bladder tumor.** UA is positive for **red blood cells (RBCs).** Cystoscopy confirms the diagnosis and allows cystoscopic resection.

c. **Bladder foreign body or stones.** UA is positive for **RBCs.** Cystoscopy confirms the diagnosis and allows cystoscopic removal.

2. **Perform a physical examination.** An examination documents any loss of pelvic support as well as intactness of neurologic innervation.

3. **Check whether cystometric parameters** are normal **(Figure 20–2).**

a. **Bladder residual volume:** < 50 ml
b. **Sensation-of-fullness volume:** 150–200 ml
c. **Urge-to-void volume:** 400–500 ml

4. Determine whether **detrusor contractions** occur with loss of urine.

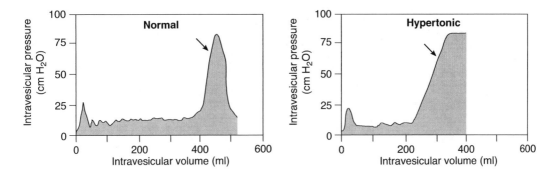

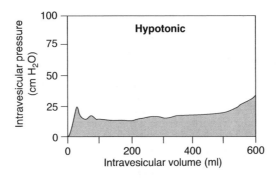

Figure 20–2. Water cystometrogram in (A) normal patient, (B) patient with hypertonic bladder, and (C) a patient with hypotonic bladder. [Redrawn with permission from Hacker NF, Moore JG (eds): *Essentials of Obstetrics and Gynecology*, 2nd ed. Philadelphia, WB Saunders, 1992, p 403.)

5. Have the patient keep a **voiding diary** to note the time of urine loss and volume of urine lost.

C. **Common types of urinary incontinence**

1. **Genuine stress incontinence** is the *most common* **cause** of incontinence in women.
   a. **Pathophysiology.** The bladder neck and proximal urethra, which are normally above the pelvic floor, lose support because of a **weak pelvic diaphragm** so they are no longer intra-abdominal.
   (1) With coughing and sneezing, increase in **intra-abdominal pressure** is transmitted more to the bladder and less to the urethra **(Figure 20–3).**
   (2) **Small amounts of urine are lost** when bladder pressure rises above urethral pressure, but **detrusor contractions do not occur.**
   b. **Clinical findings.** Evidence of pelvic relaxation may be seen (e.g., cystocele) [see I B 2].
   (1) **No urine loss occurs when the patient is sleeping. With coughing and sneezing,** loss of only **small amounts of urine** take place, with no occurrence of detrusor contractions.
   (2) **Neurologic examination is normal,** with voluntary inhibition of detrusor contractions possible.
   (3) **Cystometry is normal** (see II B 3).
   c. **Management**
   (1) **Kegel exercises** can strengthen the pelvic floor. **ERT** may improve tissue tone in postmenopausal women.

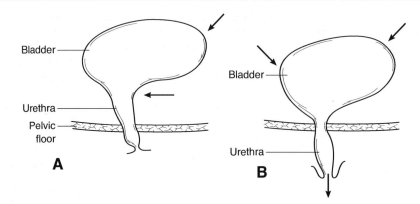

Figure 20–3. Urinary continence and incontinence are related to the transmission of intra-abdominal pressure *(arrows)* to the bladder and urethra. (A) Maintenance of urinary continence by equal transmission of abdominal pressure to the bladder and the urethra when they are in their proper anatomic locations. (B) However, abdominal pressure is transmitted only to the bladder when the urethra lies underneath the pelvic floor, thus causing a pressure increase that exceeds urethral closure pressure, resulting in urine loss. (After Clarke-Pearson DL, Dawood MY: *Green's Gynecology: Essentials of Clinical Practice,* 4th ed. Boston, Little, Brown, 1990, p 404.)

(2) Surgical elevation of the urethrovesical angle (urethropexy) is the definitive treatment. This procedure restores the normal intra-abdominal position of the proximal urethra, bladder neck, and bladder.

2. **Hypertonic, motor urge incontinence** is the second most common cause. This condition is also called unstable bladder, detrusor hyperreflexia, or detrusor dyssynergia. Incidence increases after menopause.
   a. **Pathophysiology.** Normal anatomic relationships between the bladder and proximal urethra are maintained.
      (1) The hypertonic **detrusor muscle contracts involuntarily** without inhibition. **Spontaneous detrusor contractions** may be stimulated by coughing, sneezing, or hearing running water.
      (2) When detrusor contractions occur, bladder pressure rises above urethral pressure, resulting in bladder emptying with **losses of larger volumes of urine.**
   b. **Clinical findings.** Pelvic examination is usually normal.
      (1) Urine loss occurs **both day and night.**
      (2) **Neurologic examination** is normal but spontaneous detrusor contractions occur without voluntary inhibition.
      (3) **Cystometry is abnormal** (bladder residual volume, < 75 ml; sensation-of-fullness volume, < 150 ml; urge-to-void volume, < 250 ml).
   c. **Management.** Treatment is medical. **Anticholinergic medications** [oxybutinin (Ditropan), propantheline (Pro-Banthine)] can decrease involuntary detrusor contractions. **β-Adrenergic agonists** [flavoxate (Urispas)] can increase bladder neck tone. **Nonsteroidal anti-inflammatory drugs (NSAIDs)** can inhibit detrusor contractions.

3. **Hypotonic, overflow incontinence** is a less common cause.
   a. **Pathophysiology**
      (1) The hypotonic detrusor muscle does not contract. This may be due to **neurologic disease or systemic medication** (ganglionic blockers, anticholinergics, α-adrenergic agonists, or regional anesthetics).

(2) Ongoing urine production increases bladder volume, with gradual increases in intravesical pressure. When the intravesical pressure exceeds the urethral pressure, **spontaneous loss of small amounts of urine** occurs, lasting only as long as it takes for bladder pressure to fall below the urethral pressure. However, the bladder never empties.

b. Clinical findings
  (1) Loss of small amounts of urine occurs constantly **both day and night.**
  (2) **Neurologic examination** may show a denervated bladder. Detrusor contractions do not take place.
  (3) **Cystometry is abnormal** (elevated bladder residual volume, > 500 ml; decreased bladder sensation; elevated bladder capacity, >1000 ml).

c. **Management.** Treatment is medical.
  (1) **Cholinergic medications** [bethanechol (Urecholine)] can stimulate detrusor contractility. **α-Adrenergic blockers** [phenoxybenzamine (Dibenzyline)] can decrease bladder neck tone.
  (2) **Intermittent self-catheterization** can ensure bladder emptying.

4. **Bypass incontinence** is uncommon. It results from a fistula that passes urine by an otherwise normal bladder and urethra. A **urinary tract fistula** should be considered if the patient has a history of radical pelvic surgery or radiation therapy.
  a. **Pathophysiology.** Detrusor contractions do not occur, and **urine loss is continual.**
  b. **Clinical findings. Cystometry is normal,** but a vesicle-vaginal fistula is diagnosed when an intravenous (IV) indigo– carmine dye injection identifies the location of the fistula by leaking onto a vaginal tampon.
  c. **Management. Surgical repair** is necessary.

Clinical Situation 20–1

Basic Case: A woman comes to the office complaining of pelvic pressure.

Patient Snapshot	Intervention	Clinical Pearls
She is **45 years of age** and healthy. Exam shows a **mild cystocele.**	Have the patient do Kegel exercises.	**Nonsurgical therapy** may help by strengthening the pelvic diaphragm muscles.
➥ Exam shows a **significant cystocele.**	Perform anterior colporrhaphy.	**Surgical therapy** plicates the fascia, providing support for the bladder. Excess vaginal mucosa is removed.
She is **57 years of age** and healthy. Exam shows a **mild cystocele.**	Have the patient do Kegel exercises and advise hormone replacement therapy.	**Nonsurgical therapy** that involves strengthening the pelvic diaphragm muscles may be helpful. **Estrogen** improves pelvic tissue tone.
➥ Exam shows a **significant cystocele.**	Perform anterior colporrhaphy and advise hormone replacement therapy.	**Surgical therapy** plicates the fascia, providing support for the bladder. **Estrogen** improves pelvic tissue tone.
➥ Exam shows second-degree **uterine prolapse.** She is not a surgical candidate.	Insert vaginal pessary and advise hormone replacement therapy.	A **pessary** placed in the vagina mechanically elevates the uterus into a more normal position. **Estrogen** improves pelvic tissue tone.

Clinical Situation 20–2

Basic Case: A 43-year-old woman comes to the office complaining of involuntary urine loss.

Patient Snapshot	Intervention	Clinical Pearls
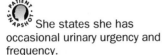 She states she has occasional urinary urgency and frequency.	Obtain urinalysis and urine culture.	**Irritative lower urinary tract lesions** (infections, tumors, foreign bodies) must first be ruled out.
➥ **Scenario 1** Loss of small amounts of urine occurs with coughing and sneezing, but not at night. Residual volume is 50 ml.	Have the patient do Kegel exercises, or perform urethropexy.	**Genuine stress incontinence** is uniquely caused by loss of support of proximal urethra. Neurologic exam is within normal limits.
➥ **Scenario 2** Loss of large amounts of urine occurs without warning day and night. Cystometry shows bladder contractions.	Use anticholinergics, NSAIDs, and anti-depressants.	**Motor urge incontinence** is uniquely caused by involuntary contractions of an uninhibited detrusor muscle.
➥ **Scenario 3** Loss of small amounts of urine occurs day and night, along with pelvic pressure. Residual volume is 450 ml.	Recommend cholinergic agents or intermittent self-catheterization.	**Overflow incontinence** occurs uniquely when intravesical pressure from an overdistended hypotonic bladder exceeds urethral pressure.
➥ **Scenario 4** Loss of urine occurs continuously day and night. She has a history of pelvic radiation. IV indigo–carmine dye leaks onto vaginal tampons.	Perform surgical repair of vesicovaginal fistula.	**Bypass incontinence** occurs uniquely when the normal urethral sphincteric mechanism is bypassed by a fistula often due to radiation or radical surgery.

IV = intravenous   NSAIDs = nonsteroidal anti-inflammatory drug

21

Enlarged Uterus

I. PREGNANCY. This condition is the *most common* cause of an enlarged uterus in the reproductive years. Pregnancy should be ruled out with **qualitative β-human chorionic gonadotropin (β-hCG) testing.**

II. LEIOMYOMAS. These myomas are the *most common* uterine tumors. Prevalence is highest in multiparous women in their fifth decade of life. **Black women are five times more likely** to develop myomas than white women.

  A. Structure and pathophysiology. Uterine myomas are **benign smooth muscle tumors.**

  1. Leiomyomas may be single, but most are multiple.

  2. These tumors may vary in size from microscopic to massive, with weights of up to 50 pounds.

  3. Myomas, which have high concentrations of both **estrogen and progesterone receptors,** often increase in size during pregnancy and involute following menopause.

  B. Types. Leiomyomas are classified based on their anatomic relationship to the uterus as well as their location within the myometrium **(Figure 21–1).**

  1. The three most common types are:
  a. Intramural (within the uterine wall)
  b. Subserous (deforming the external serosa)
  c. Submucous (deforming the uterine cavity)

  2. These tumors may have a wide base or be **pedunculated,** with a narrow stalk. Such tumors are seldom within the uterine cavity.

  C. Symptoms. Most intramural and subserous myomas are **asymptomatic.**

  1. Submucous myomas are associated with **abnormal menstrual bleeding** and second-trimester pregnancy loss.

  2. Large myomas can produce **pressure effects.**

  3. Rapid myoma growth during pregnancy can result in acute infarction, causing **severe pain or carneous degeneration.**

  D. Examination. The uterus is usually **enlarged, firm, nontender,** and **asymmetrical.**

  E. Imaging studies. A **hysterosalpingogram (HSG)** or **hysteroscopy** can be used to identify submucous myomas. **Sonography** or **magnetic resonance imaging (MRI)** allows visualization of intramural or submucous myomas.

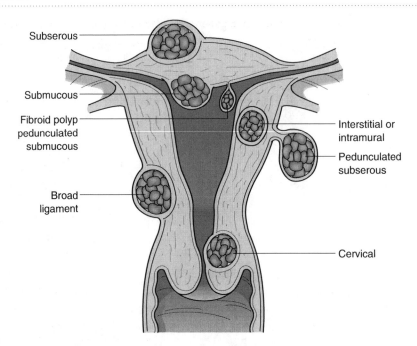

Figure 21–1. Common types of uterine leiomyomas. (After Beckmann CR, Ling FW, Barzansky BM et al: *Obstetrics and Gynecology*, 2nd ed. Baltimore, Williams & Wilkins, 1995, p 440.)

F. Management

1. **Conservative management** is appropriate for most patients with myomas, unless the tumors are symptomatic. Steroid therapy can cause leiomyomas to enlarge.

2. **Embolization.** This is an interventional radiology procedure where uterine artery catheters are placed under fluoroscopy through the femoral approach. Polyvinyl alcohol (PVA) microspheres are then injected to cause ischemia, necrosis, and devascularization of the leiomyomas. Significant decreases in leiomyoma size are expected. Inadvertent ovarian artery embolization rarely can occur. If a pregnancy subsequently occurs, higher rates of premature birth, cesarean section, and postpartum hemorrhage are reported.

3. **Surgery** may be necessary. **Hysterectomy** is the only definitive cure. **Hysteroscopic resection** of intracavitary myomas can be effective. **Surgical myomectomy** can remove large or multiple symptomatic myomas after preoperative shrinkage with gonadotropin-releasing hormone (GnRH) agonists. However, recurrence is common.

III. ADENOMYOSIS. Prevalence is highest in multiparous women during the fourth and fifth decades of life.

A. Pathophysiology. Endometrial glands and stroma are found within the myometrial wall, possibly resulting in cyclic bleeding into the myometrium. Involvement may be diffuse throughout the myometrium or localized into an **adenomyoma.**

B. Symptoms

1. **Symptom severity** is proportional to the depth of myometrial penetration and uterine size. Most affected patients have minor symptoms or are asymptomatic.

2. Secondary dysmenorrhea or abnormal menstrual bleeding usually develops.

C. **Examination.** The uterus is usually enlarged, **soft, tender,** and **symmetrical.**

D. **Imaging studies.** Sonography or MRI imaging may be helpful if the lesion is severe or diffuse.

E. **Management.** No medical management has proved effective. **Hysterectomy is the only definitive cure.**

IV. LEIOMYOSARCOMAS

A. **Pathophysiology.** Leiomyosarcomas are **malignant smooth muscle tumors** of the uterus. **Most tumors probably arise de novo** rather than from malignant transformation of preexisting myomas.

B. **Symptoms. Most affected patients have no symptoms** initially. Later, pain and vaginal bleeding develop.

C. **Examination.** The uterus is enlarged and growing rapidly.

D. **Management.** Surgical exploration followed by total abdominal hysterectomy and bilateral salpingo-oophorectomy (TAH-BSO) is imperative. Chemotherapy and radiation therapy are only adjunctive.

E. **Prognosis.** The outcome worsens with vascular invasion, extrauterine spread, and increasing mitosis count per high-power field.

22

Endometrial Hyperplasia and Cancer

I. ENDOMETRIAL HYPERPLASIA

A. Epidemiology: risk factors

   1. **Prolonged estrogen exposure:** nulliparity, late menopause, chronic unopposed estrogen, tamoxifen (paradoxical effect of this antiestrogen)

   2. **Systemic diseases:** diabetes mellitus (DM), chronic hypertension, obesity

   3. **Other cancers:** breast, colon, ovarian

B. **Pathophysiology. Unopposed estrogen stimulation** (without progesterone ripening followed by withdrawal bleeding) is the *most common* cause of endometrial hyperplasia. The hyperplasia may be **generalized,** involving the entire endometrium, or may be **localized,** involving only focal areas. **Histology** may vary from mild to severe.

   1. **Simple and cystic hyperplasia,** involving both glandular and stromal elements, very rarely progresses to cancer.

   2. **Complex hyperplasia WITHOUT atypia** (involving only glandular elements), usually also remains benign.

   3. **Complex hyperplasia WITH atypia** progresses to endometrial carcinoma in one-third of cases.

C. Clinical findings

   1. **Symptoms** include abnormal vaginal bleeding.

   2. **Pelvic examination** is usually normal.

   3. **Diagnosis** is by **endometrial biopsy.**

D. Management

   1. **Cyclic progestins** reverse most hyperplasias without atypia. A trial of progestins is also appropriate in premenopausal women with atypical hyperplasia desiring fertility preservation.

   2. Follow-up **biopsies** should be performed in 3–6 months.

   3. **Total hysterectomy** is appropriate for atypical hyperplasia in all postmenopausal women and premenopausal women who have completed childbearing.

II. ENDOMETRIAL CANCER

A. Epidemiology

1. This is the *most common* **gynecologic malignancy,** with average age at diagnosis of **61 years.** The *most common* **tumor type** is **adenocarcinoma** (75% of cases). Less common types are adenosquamous carcinoma and clear cell carcinoma.

2. No formal **screening** test exists. Abnormal bleeding is followed by endometrial tissue sampling. Most tumors are diagnosed at an early stage and low grade, leading to a **favorable outcome.**

3. Risk factors are the same as those for endometrial hyperplasia (see I A).

B. Pathophysiology. Endometrial stimulation by **unopposed estrogen** leads to endometrial cancer. Atypical complex hyperplasia is the precursor to endometrial carcinoma. The *most common* **route of primary spread** involves direct extension to the myometrium and cervix.

1. Transtubal spread occurs to the ovaries, peritoneum, and omentum.

2. Lymphatic spread occurs from the pelvic to the periaortic nodes.

C. Clinical findings

1. Symptoms. Postmenopausal bleeding is the *most common* symptom.

2. Examination. Pelvic examination is usually normal, with uterine enlargement seen only in advanced disease.

3. Diagnosis. A definitive diagnosis can be made only by tissue histology using fractional dilation and curettage (D&C) and hysteroscopy.

a. Fractional D&C obtains two separate specimens. An endocervical curettage (ECC) is performed first to assess for metastasis to the cervix. This is followed by dilation of the cervical canal to allow hysteroscopy, and then the endometrial curettage is performed.

Table 22–1
Surgical Staging of Endometrial Carcinoma

FIGO Stage*	Description
Stage I	**Limited to the uterus**
Ia	Limited to endometrium
Ib	Invasion less than half of myometrium
Ic	Invasion over half of myometrium
Stage II	**Limited extension beyond uterus**
IIa	Endocervical gland involvement only
IIb	Cervical stromal invasion
Stage III	**Extension within pelvis**
IIIa	Invasion of serosa/adnexa or positive peritoneal cytology
IIIb	Vaginal metastases
IIIc	Metastasis to pelvic/para-aortic nodes
Stage IV	**Distant metastases**
IVa	Invasion of bladder/bowel mucosa
IVb	Distant metastases/extra-abdominal or inguinal nodes

FIGO = International Federation of Gynecology and Obstetrics
*Tumors are also further defined according to their histology as grade 1, 2, or 3.

   b. **Hysteroscopy** is performed after the ECC of the fractional D&C. It identifies abnormal-appearing tissue and allows directed biopsy of **localized lesions** such as endometrial polyps.

D. **Staging (Table 22–1).** Note that staging is performed surgically.

E. **Management**

   1. **Total abdominal hysterectomy and bilateral salpingo-oophorectomy (TAH-BSO)** is the basic treatment for all stages.

   2. **Specific management** is determined by cancer stage.
   a. **Stage I** is managed with a TAH-BSO.
   b. **Stage II** is managed with preoperative radiation followed by TAH-BSO.
   c. **Stages III and IV** are managed with TAH-BSO, radiation therapy, progestins, and chemotherapy.

Clinical Situation 22–1

Basic Case: A woman comes to the office with 6 months of abnormal menstrual bleeding.

Patient Snapshot	Intervention	Clinical Pearls
She is **30 years of age.** The bleeding is unpredictable and irregular. Her weight is 180 lb and her height is 5'3." Her BP is 155/90 mm Hg. Her β-hCG is negative.	Perform endometrial biopsy.	Even though she is young, her **obesity** and **HTN** place her at higher risk for atypical hyperplasia. Endometrial biopsy is essential.
➡ 3 days later: Endometrial biopsy indicates complex hyperplasia **without atypia.**	Recommend progestin cycling. Repeat biopsy in 3–6 months.	Hormonal management is the treatment of choice. Complex hyperplasia **without atypia** has a **high rate of reversal** with 3–6 months of progestin cycling.
She is **42 years of age** with a FBS of 140 mg/dl. The bleeding is unpredictable and irregular. Her weight is 180 lb, and her height is 5'3." Her BP is 155/90 mm Hg. Her urine β-hCG is negative.	Perform endometrial biopsy.	Her unpredictable bleeding suggests **anovulation,** which along with her **age, diabetes, obesity,** and **HTN,** yields many risk factors for endometrial CA. It is essential to rule out atypical hyperplasia or CA.
➡ 3 days later: The pathology report on the endometrial biopsy shows complex hyperplasia **with atypia.**	Perform total hysterectomy (vaginal or abdominal).	Surgery is the treatment of choice. Complex hyperplasia **with atypia** is the precursor to endometrial carcinoma. It has a **low rate of reversal** with progestin therapy.

BP = blood pressure   FBS = fasting blood sugar   HTN = hypertension
CA = carcinoma   hCG = human chorionic gonadotropin

Clinical Situation 22–2

Basic Case: A 59-year-old $G_3P_3A_0$ postmenopausal woman comes to the office with a history of 2 weeks of painless vaginal bleeding. She is not taking any hormonal replacement therapy.

Patient Snapshot	Intervention	Clinical Pearls
Her weight is 135 lb, and her height is 5'5." Her BP is 130/75 mm Hg. She has a history of breast cancer and is taking **tamoxifen.**	Perform hysteroscopy and fractional D&C after ruling out GI and lower reproductive tract causes.	She is not obese or hypertensive, but **tamoxifen** is a risk factor with an endometrial **estrogen agonist** effect. A tissue diagnosis is imperative.
➥ 3 days later: Endometrial biopsy indicates complex hyperplasia **with atypia.**	Perform total hysterectomy (vaginal or abdominal).	Surgery is the treatment of choice. Complex hyperplasia **with atypia** is the precursor to endometrial carcinoma. It has a **low rate of reversal** with progestin therapy.
Her weight is 180 lb and her height is 5'3." Her BP is 155/90 mm Hg. She has prominent facial hair. She required ovulation induction for her pregnancies.	Perform hysteroscopy and fractional D&C after ruling out GI and lower reproductive tract causes.	The clinical picture is that of PCO syndrome. **Anovulation, diabetes, obesity,** and **HTN** are clear risk factors for endometrial CA. A tissue diagnosis is imperative.
➥ 3 days later: The pathology report shows grade 1 endometrial CA with cervical glandular involvement.	Order preoperative pelvic radiation and perform staging laparotomy with TAH-BSO.	Because of the metastasis to the cervix, this case is **at least stage II,** with a resulting increased risk of lymphatic invasion. Therefore, **preoperative pelvic radiation** is indicated.

BP = blood pressure	GI = gastrointestinal	PCO = polycystic ovarian syndrome
CA = carcinoma	HTN = hypertension	TAH-BSO = total abdominal hysterectomy and
D&C = dilation and curettage		bilateral salpingo-oophorectomy

23

Ovarian Neoplasia and Cancer

I. BENIGN OVARIAN NEOPLASIA

A. Origin of pelvic masses. Three organ systems are located within the pelvis, and they should all be considered as possible sources of pelvic masses.

  1. **Reproductive tract** sources are the uterus, oviducts, and ovaries.

  2. **Urinary tract** sources include pelvic kidneys, ureteroceles, and renal tumors.

  3. **Gastrointestinal (GI)** tract sources include colorectal tumors and diverticulosis.

B. Types of benign premenopausal ovarian masses

  1. **Functional masses,** which result from an excessive response to otherwise normal reproductive events, are the *most common* **type** of premenopausal ovarian cystic mass.

   a. **Follicular cysts** are **unilateral** and resolve within 60 days.

   b. **Corpus luteum cysts** are **unilateral** and resolve within 60 days. They are often associated with pregnancy.

   c. **Theca lutein cysts** are **bilateral,** associated with high β-human chorionic gonadotropin (β-hCG) titers, and may take months to resolve.

  2. **Nonfunctional, nonneoplastic masses** arise neither from normal reproductive events nor neoplastic processes.

   a. **Endometriomas,** which are called **"chocolate cysts,"** are usually **unilateral** and can be up to 10 cm in size (see Figure 17–3). The *most common* site of endometriosis is the ovary.

   b. **Polycystic ovaries** are **bilateral;** smooth and mildly enlarged to palpation; and associated with hirsutism, anovulation, and infertility.

   c. **Hyperthecosis-enlarged ovaries** are usually **bilateral** and found in middle-aged women. They produce gradually increasing amounts of androgens, leading to hirsutism and even virilization.

  3. **Neoplastic masses** are derived from benign neoplastic processes.

   a. **Serous cystadenomas** are unilocular and may become massive. These lesions are the *most common* **ovarian epithelial tumors.**

   b. **Mucinous cystadenomas** are multilocular, and if they rupture, they can result in **pseudomyxoma peritonei.**

   c. **Benign cystic teratomas,** which may contain any combination of germ layers, are often mobile on long pedicles. The *most common* **ovarian germ cell tumors,** these masses are the *most common* **ovarian neoplasms** in women less than 30 years of age.

C. Clinical approach

1. **Pregnancy,** the *most common* **cause** of premenopausal pelvic masses, **must first be ruled out** by obtaining a β-hCG test.

2. **Ovarian etiology** can be determined in three ways.
   a. Pelvic sonography, which rules out nonovarian reproductive tract origin
   b. Intravenous pyelography (IVP), which rules out urinary tract origin
   c. Barium enema, which rules out lower GI tract origin

3. **Functional ovarian etiology** (see I B 1)
   a. On **sonography,** these cysts appear unilateral, mobile, simple, and fluid-filled.
   b. Management of follicular or corpus luteum cysts involves **observation** for 30–60 days. If the masses regress, no further follow-up is needed. **Surgical evaluation** is necessary for persistent masses.
   c. Management of theca lutein cysts or pregnancy luteomas involves **observation,** looking for spontaneous regression after pregnancy.

4. **Nonfunctional ovarian masses** should be evaluated surgically using one of the techniques listed below.
   a. Laparoscopy is appropriate if a **benign mass** is suspected.
   b. Laparotomy is appropriate if a **malignant mass** is suspected.
   c. Sonographically guided cyst aspiration is **controversial,** because a malignant cyst could rupture, seeding the peritoneal cavity.

5. **Ovarian torsion** must always be considered, regardless of tumor etiology.
   a. Risk factors include large size (> 6–8 cm) and mobility.
   b. Symptoms include sudden onset of acute, unilateral pelvic pain with rebound abdominal tenderness.
   c. Management involves emergency laparotomy to prevent ischemic injury to the ovary.

6. **Malignancy screening** is based on ultrasound and examination findings.
   a. Benign tumors are more likely to have smooth, regular surfaces and be mobile, unilateral, small, and simple.
   b. Malignant tumors are more likely to have nodular or irregular surfaces and be fixed, bilateral, large, complex, or loculated.

II. OVARIAN CANCER

A. Epidemiology

1. **Prevalence.** This type of cancer is the **second most common gynecologic malignancy (25%),** with a mean age at diagnosis of 69 years (higher than all other gynecologic malignancies.)

2. **Risk factors.** Predisposing factors include **BRCA1 gene, positive family history,** greater lifetime ovulations (i.e., nulliparity, infertility, late menopause), Caucasian or Asian ethnicity, perineal talc use, and older age (> age 60 years).

3. **Screening.** Annual **bimanual pelvic examination** is used to detect abnormal pelvic masses.

B. Pathophysiology

1. **Tumor type.** The *most common* tumor type is **epithelial** (80%), followed by **germ cell** (15%), and **gonadal stromal** (5%). Epithelial carcinomas may originate from serial disruptions of the ovarian germinal capsule as a result of repeated ovulations.

2. **Route of spread.** The *most common* route of primary spread is by **implantation of exfoliated cells** via peritoneal fluid circulation involving the omentum, cul-de-sac, paracolic gutters, and liver capsule. Lymphatic spread occurs from the superficial to the deep inguinal nodes.

3. **Origin. Metastatic tumors,** which are usually **bilateral,** may originate from the breast, GI tract, or endometrium.

C. Clinical findings

1. **Symptoms. Early disease** is nearly always **asymptomatic,** unless the tumor has produced hormones such as estrogens or androgens. **Advanced disease** tends to result **in nonspecific symptoms** such as nausea, change in bowel habits, and early satiety.

2. **Examination.** Pelvic and abdominal masses that are fixed, bilateral, and nodular are suggestive of ovarian cancer. Abdominal distention and ascites are found with advanced spread.

3. **Diagnosis.** Definitive diagnosis can be made only by **histologic examination** of the removed ovary or malignant tissue.

D. Tumor markers

1. **Epithelial tumors: cancer antigen 125 (CA-125)** and **carcinogenic embryonic antigen (CEA)**

2. Germ cell tumors: α-fetoprotein (AFP), β-hCG, lactate dehydrogenase (LDH)

3. Gonadal-stromal tumors: **estrogen** and **testosterone**

E. Staging (Table 23–1). Note that **staging is performed surgically.** Most cases are diagnosed at stage III, with widespread peritoneal spread and subsequently poor prognosis.

Table 23–1
Surgical Staging of Ovarian Carcinoma

FIGO Stage	Description
Stage I	**Limited to the ovaries**
Ia	Limited to one ovary; no malignant ascites; capsule intact
Ib	Limited to both ovaries; no malignant ascites; capsule intact
Ic	Limited to ovaries; malignant ascites present; capsule not intact
Stage II	**Limited extension beyond ovaries**
IIa	Extension to uterus/tubes
IIb	Extension to other pelvic tissues
IIc	IIa or IIb with malignant ascites or positive peritoneal washings
Stage III	**Extension within the pelvis**
IIIa	Limited to true pelvis; negative nodes; positive peritoneal seeding
IIIb	Same as IIIa, but implants < 2 cm diameter
IIIc	Same as IIIa, but implants > 2 cm diameter and/or positive nodes
Stage IV	**Distant metastases**
	Distant metastases, pleural effusion, or parenchymal liver metastases

FIGO = International Federation of Gynecology and Obstetrics

F. Management. Basic treatment for all stages of ovarian cancer involves total abdominal hysterectomy and bilateral salpingo-oophorectomy (TAH-BSO) and omentectomy.

1. Unilateral salpingo-oophorectomy is appropriate only for stage Ia cancer in young women who wish to preserve fertility.

2. Radiation therapy is adjunctive for all patients.

3. Cytoreductive debulking surgery is indicated for advanced cancer that has spread diffusely in the peritoneal cavity.

Clinical Situation 23–1

Basic Case: A 25-year-old woman comes to the office for a routine visit, complaining of pelvic pressure. On pelvic exam you note a pelvic mass.

Patient Snapshot	Intervention	Clinical Pearls
The mass is 5 cm in size, freely mobile, nontender, and smooth to palpation.	Obtain qualitative β-hCG test and pelvic sonogram.	A **pregnant uterus** can be deviated from the midline, presenting as an adnexal mass.
Scenario 1 She is not pregnant and is using a **diaphragm** for contraception. You feel a 5-cm **cystic** adnexal mass that is confirmed by sonography.	Observe and perform repeat exam in 6 weeks.	This is most likely a **functional cyst** (follicular or corpus luteum) that will spontaneously regress.
Scenario 2 She is not pregnant and is using a **diaphragm** for contraception. You feel a 5-cm **solid** adnexal mass that is confirmed by sonography.	Perform pelvic laparoscopy.	This is probably a **neoplastic mass** that must be surgically removed. Functional masses are never solid.
Scenario 3 She is not pregnant and is using **OCPs** for contraception. You feel a 5-cm cystic adnexal mass that is confirmed by sonography.	Perform pelvic laparoscopy.	This is probably a **neoplastic mass** that must be removed. OCPs should suppress FSH and LH; thus, functional cysts should not develop.
She is 8 weeks **pregnant** after ovulation induction. A sonogram shows **bilateral** 7-cm adnexal masses, which are partially solid and partially cystic.	Observe.	**Theca lutein cysts** are the response of normal ovaries to ↑ β-hCG levels. Spontaneous resolution occurs but may take months.
She is not pregnant but has a known unilateral 9-cm cystic pelvic mass. She now complains of **sudden RLQ pain.**	Perform emergency exploratory laparotomy.	**Ovarian torsion** is a true emergency in which delay in restoring blood supply could result in ovarian infarction.

FSH = follicle-stimulating hormone   LH = luteinizing hormone   RLQ = right lower quadrant
β-hCG = β-human chorionic gonadotropin   OCP = oral contraceptive pill

Clinical Situation 23–2

Patient Snapshot	Intervention	Clinical Pearls
A 55-year-old woman comes to the outpatient office complaining of pelvic pressure and abdominal fullness. Her LMP was 3 years ago.	Perform thorough general and pelvic exam.	**Ovarian CA** must be suspected. The screening method of choice is a thorough pelvic exam.
➤ On exam you find a left adnexal mass that is 5-cm in diameter and **cystic** to palpation. Your findings are confirmed by sonography.	Obtain BE and IVP, and then perform staging exploratory laparotomy.	Assume ovarian CA. Even though it is cystic, this mass **cannot be functional.** Because no functioning follicles exist, follicular or corpus luteum cysts are not possible.
➤ On exam you find a left adnexal mass that is 5-cm in diameter and **solid** to palpation. Your findings are confirmed by sonography.	Obtain BE and IVP, and then perform staging exploratory laparotomy.	**Ovarian malignancy** must be ruled out. Functional masses are never solid.
➤ **Scenario 1** BE and IVP are normal. Staging exploratory laparotomy is performed. You find **stage Ia** ovarian CA.	Perform TAH-BSO and infracolic omentectomy.	Histology suggests the CA is confined to the ovary, but the 5-year survival rate is only 80%.
➤ **Scenario 2** BE and IVP are normal. Staging exploratory laparotomy is performed. You find **stage II** ovarian CA.	Perform TAH-BSO and infracolic omentectomy, but also use chemotherapy.	All patients with ovarian CA beyond stage Ia should also receive **chemotherapy.**
➤ **Scenario 3** BE and IVP are normal. Staging exploratory laparotomy is performed. You find **stage III** ovarian CA.	Perform TAH-BSO and infracolic omentectomy, with chemotherapy, but also use cytoreductive debulking.	With advanced ovarian CA, the aim is to leave **no residual tumor** nodules > 1.5 cm.

BE = barium enema   IVP = intravenous pyelogram   TAH-BSO = total abdominal hysterectomy
CA = carcinoma   LMP = last menstrual period   and bilateral salpingo-oophorectomy

Clinical Situation 23–3

Patient Snapshot	Intervention	Clinical Pearls
A 26-year-old woman who is G_1P_1 is diagnosed with **well-differentiated stage Ia** ovarian serous cystadenocarcinoma. She wants more children.	Perform unilateral SO (no hysterectomy).	This is the only situation in which conservative management may be appropriate.
A 26-year-old woman who is G_1P_1 is diagnosed with **well-differentiated stage II** ovarian serous cystadenocarcinoma. She wants more children.	Perform TAH-BSO and infracolic omentectomy.	Conservative management is inappropriate once the CA has spread beyond the ovary.
A 36-year-old woman who is G_4P_4 is diagnosed with **well-differentiated stage Ia** ovarian serous cystadenocarcinoma.	Perform TAH-BSO and infracolic omentectomy.	Even with localized stage Ia CA, if childbearing is completed, the risk of recurrence is high enough to justify aggressive surgery.

CA = carcinoma   SO = salpingo-oophorectomy   TAH-BSO = total abdominal hysterectomy and bilateral salpingo-oophorectomy

24

Cervical Neoplasia and Cancer

I. CERVICAL INTRAEPITHELIAL NEOPLASIA (CIN)

A. Pathophysiology. CIN arises from the **transformation zone** (T-zone) of the cervix, where human papilloma virus (HPV), especially types 16 and 18, may alter the normal metaplasia of columnar epithelium to squamous epithelium **(Figure 24–1)**. Intraepithelial refers to the abnormal, immature, disorganized dysplastic cells contained **within** the epithelium, with the basement membrane intact.

   1. **CIN** 1 is the histological diagnosis when dysplastic cells occupy the lower third of the epithelium (**mild** dysplasia).

   2. **CIN** 2 is the histological diagnosis when dysplastic cells occupy up to the middle third of the epithelium.

   3. **CIN** 3 is the histological diagnosis when dysplastic cells extend into the upper third and may occupy the full thickness of the epithelium.

B. Natural history. Most mild dysplasia will spontaneously **resolve** (65%), some remain **static** (20%) but others will **progress** (15%) through to severe dysplasia and carcinoma-in-situ (CIS) **(Chart 24–1).**

C. Risk factors. Early age of coitus, multiple sexual partners, cigarette smoking, immunosuppression, and genital infection with **HPV,** especially types **16 and 18. Oral contraceptive** use (especially over 10 years duration) is associated with cervical adenocarcinoma. CIN is found in association with vulvar intraepithelial neoplasia (VIN).

D. Pap smear cytological screening methods. Cells from the exocervical T-zone and endocervical canal are obtained and examined cytologically for neoplastic changes.

   1. Conventional method. Cytological specimens are obtained by scraping the exocervix with a spatula and the endocervical cervical canal with a brush. The specimen is smeared on a glass slide, stabilized with a fixative, then microscopically examined by a cytologist. Disadvantages include false negative results from abnormal cells discarded by remaining on the collection device and abnormal cells obscured on the slide because of blood and pus as well as non-uniform distribution on the slide.

   2. Thin-layer, liquid-based cytology changes the way cell samples are placed on a slide and prepared for analysis. The cell collection device is rinsed into a vial of preserving solution, which is sent to the lab for purification of debris. The remaining cells are deposited on a slide as a thin layer of processed cells. Advantages include minimized loss of abnormal cells on the collection device and more

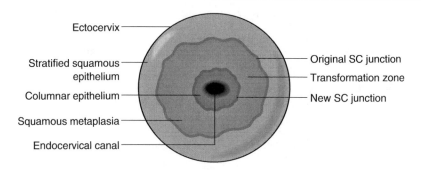

Ectocervix

Stratified squamous epithelium

Columnar epithelium

Squamous metaplasia

Endocervical canal

Original SC junction

Transformation zone

New SC junction

Figure 24–1.   Development of the transformation (T) zone of the cervix between the original squamo-columnar (SC) junction and the new SC junction.

uniform cell distribution on the slide. HPV DNA testing can also be performed on the specimen.

3. **Computer-assisted automated cytology** uses high-speed video microscopy and image interpretation software to screen conventionally prepared Pap smears and indicate which slides to screen manually.

4. **Hybrid Capture 2 HPV DNA testing** uses signal amplification and immuno capture of DNA hybrids of the 13 most frequent oncogenic HPV types in cervical samples obtained either separately by cytobrush or simultaneously on the liquid-based cytology collection vial.

E. **Timing of Pap smear screening**

1. **Initiate screening** within 3 years of onset of vaginal intercourse or no later than age 21.

Natural History of Cervical Dysplasia
Response to HPV Types

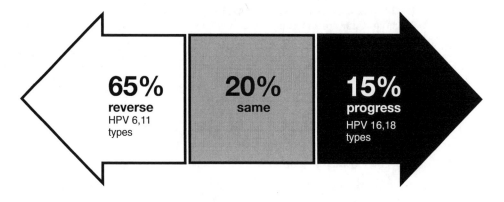

65%
reverse
HPV 6,11 types

20%
same

15%
progress
HPV 16,18 types

HPV = human papillomavirus

Chart 24–1.

2. **Stop screening** at age 70 if the patient has had 3 or more consecutive normal Pap smears.

3. **After total hysterectomy** (cervix removed), vaginal cuff Pap smears are not indicated if the procedure was performed for benign disease.

4. **After subtotal hysterectomy** (with cervix intact), continue usual Pap smears as per recommendations.

F. **Frequency of Pap smear screening**

1. **Age under 30.** Perform annually with conventional methods or every 2 years using liquid-based cytology.

2. **Age 30 or over.** Screen every 2 to 3 years if 3 or more consecutive normal annual Pap smears.

G. **Pap smear reporting (2001 Bethesda System)** should include:

1. **Statement regarding adequacy.** The specimen is either **satisfactory** for evaluation or **unsatisfactory** in which case the reason should be specified. If the Pap smear is unsatisfactory, it should be repeated in 6–12 weeks.

2. **Statement regarding interpretation/result.** If the specimen is other than negative, the epithelial cell abnormality should be specified:

   a. **Negative for intraepithelial lesion or malignancy.** This is the desired statement. It may also include comments regarding inflammation, organisms (e.g., trichomoniasis, yeast, herpes), or atrophy.

   b. **Squamous epithelial cell abnormalities.** This may include any one of the following:

      (1) **Atypical squamous cells (ASCs),** which are divided into **ASC-US** (ASC of uncertain significance) or **ASC-H** (ASC cannot exclude high-grade lesion).

      (2) **Low-grade squamous intraepithelial lesion (LSIL)** consistent with changes of a transient HPV infection unlikely to progress to cancer. This encompasses HPV, mild dysplasia, and CIN 1.

      (3) **High-grade squamous intraepithelial lesion (HSIL)** consistent with changes due to HPV viral persistence and higher suspicion for invasive potential. This encompasses moderate/severe dysplasia/CIS and CIN 2/CIN 3.

      (4) **Cancer** consistent with invasive malignant squamous carcinoma.

   c. **Glandular epithelial cell abnormalities.** These are often of endocervical (EC) or endometrial (EM) origin and may include any one of the following:

      (1) **AGC-benign (atypical glandular cells)** from EC or EM origin favoring a **benign** nature.

      (2) **AGC-NOS (atypical glandular cells not otherwise specified)** favoring a benign nature.

      (3) **AGC-neoplastic** favoring a **neoplastic** nature.

      (4) **Endocervical adenocarcinoma in situ (AIS)**

      (5) **Cancer** consistent with invasive malignant adenocarcinoma.

H. **Pap smear followup procedures**

1. **Accelerated repeat Pap** is one option for **ASC-US.** Repeat Pap at 4- to 6-month intervals until two consecutive negative Paps. If a second Pap is ASC-US or worse, refer for colposcopy.

2. **HPV DNA testing** is a second option for **ASC-US** sending residual cells from the initial liquid-based Pap for HPV DNA testing. If the initial ASC-US Pap smear

was conventional, a second Pap could be performed by also obtaining an HPV DNA sample. The HPV specimen is sent for DNA testing only if the repeat Pap again comes back as ASC-US.

3. **Colposcopy** of the cervix is a third option with **ASC-US** but it is always performed for Pap smears that show squamous cell abnormalities (**ASC-H, LSIL, HSIL,** or **cancer**) or any glandular cell abnormalities (**AGC** or **AIS**).
   a. **Satisfactory** or **adequate colposcopy** is diagnosed if the entire T-zone is visualized and no lesions disappear into the endocervical canal.
   b. **Unsatisfactory** or **inadequate** is diagnosed if the entire T-zone cannot be fully visualized.

4. **Biopsy** of abnormal cervical epithelium (**mosaicism, punctation, white epithelium** or **abnormal vessels**) is performed. The cervix is painted with acetic acid to highlight these lesions.

5. **Endocervical curettage (ECC)** is performed (to screen for an unseen lesion) if part of the T-zone extends into the endocervical canal.

6. **Diagnostic cone biopsy** is performed (to identify or clarify questionable histology) with the following indications (**Figure 24–2, left**):
   a. ECC histology shows abnormal cells.
   b. Colposcopy shows a lesion extending into the endocervical canal.
   c. Cervical biopsy shows histological changes less severe than expected by the Pap smear (**Chart 24–2**).
   d. Cervical biopsy shows either microinvasive squamous cell carcinoma or adenocarcinoma in situ.

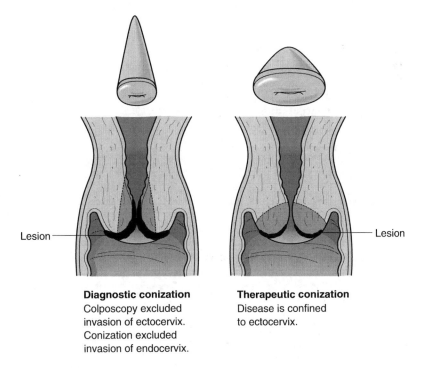

Lesion

Diagnostic conization
Colposcopy excluded
invasion of ectocervix.
Conization excluded
invasion of endocervix.

Lesion

Therapeutic conization
Disease is confined
to ectocervix.

Figure 24–2.   The extent of the tissue excised in cone biopsy depends on where disease is found. The black area represents the lesion, and the hatched area represents the tissue removed by conization.

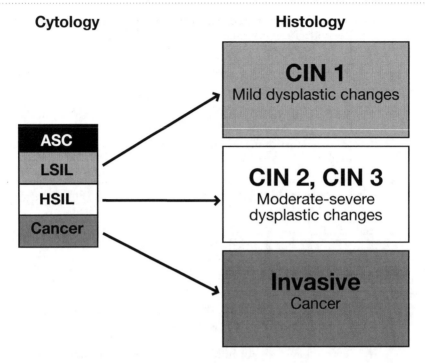

Cytology   **Histology**

CIN 1
Mild dysplastic changes

ASC
LSIL
HSIL
Cancer

CIN 2, CIN 3
Moderate-severe
dysplastic changes

Invasive
Cancer

The biopsy histology should match the Pap smear cytology.

ASC = atypical squamous cells; CIN = cervical intraepithelial neoplasia;
HSIL = high grade squamous intraepithelial lesion; LSIL = low grade squamous
epithelial lesion

Chart 24–2.

I. Management options after biopsy-confirmed CIN

   1. Observation and follow-up without treatment may be used with biopsy-confirmed **CIN 1** with satisfactory colposcopy. (Observation is never acceptable with CIN 2 or CIN 3.) Any of the following conservative approaches are acceptable:
     a. Repeat Pap smear in 6 and 12 months.
     b. Perform colposcopy and repeat Pap in 12 months.
     c. HPV DNA testing in 12 months. Observation is never acceptable with **CIN 2** or **CIN 3.**

   2. Ablative modalities include **cryotherapy** (freezing the ectocervix with liquid nitrogen), **laser** vaporization, and **electrofulguration.** ECC should be performed prior to ablation to rule out occult invasive cancer. Ablation can be used for primary treatment of **CIN 1, 2, 3. The entire transformation zone should be ablated if the biopsy showed CIN 2, 3.**

   3. Diagnostic excisional procedure includes **loop electrosurgical excision procedure (LEEP),** which uses a heated wire loop to excise lesions of the T-zone or **cold-knife conization.** These procedures should be used whenever colposcopy is unsatisfactory. They can be used for primary treatment of **CIN 1, 2, 3** and are the preferred methods for recurrent CIN after ablation procedures. **The entire transformation zone should be excised if the biopsy showed CIN 2, 3 (Figure 24–2, right).**

4. **Hysterectomy** is never acceptable for primary therapy for CIN 2, 3. It is only acceptable with biopsy-confirmed recurrent CIN 2, 3.

5. **Follow-up** is essential after ablative or excisional procedures. Options include: repeat Pap smears, colposcopy and Pap smear, or HPV DNA testing every 4–6 months.

II. CERVICAL CANCER

A. Overview

1. This is the **third most common** gynecologic malignancy (20%) with youngest average age at diagnosis—45 years.

2. The *most common* **tumor** (90%) is **squamous** type arising from the exocervix.

3. Much less common is **adenocarcinoma** arising from the endocervical columnar epithelium.

4. This is the only gynecologic cancer that is staged clinically, rather than surgically.

B. **Pathophysiology.** Invasive carcinoma occurs when the abnormal cells penetrate the basement membrane.

C. Epidemiology

1. **Screening** uses cervical Pap smear screening as described under CIN.

2. **Risk factors.** Early age of coitus, multiple sex partners, cigarette smoking, immunosuppression, and infection with **HPV** (especially types **16 and 18**)

3. **Route of spread.** Primary spread is by **direct extension.**

4. **Staging. (See Table 24–1.)** Note this is the only gynecological cancer that is **clinically** staged.

D. Clinical findings

1. **Symptoms.** Early disease is asymptomatic, but **post-coital bleeding** is the *most common* **symptom.**

Table 24–1
Clinical Staging of Cervical Carcinoma

FIGO Stage	Description
Stage 0	**Carcinoma-in-situ;** confined to the epithelium
Stage I	**Invasion is strictly confined to the cervix.**
IA1	Minimal microscopically evident stromal invasion < 3 mm deep
IA2	Microscopic invasion ≤ 5 mm, with horizontal spread ≤ 7 mm
IB	All others
Stage II	**Invasion is beyond the cervix but not to pelvic wall or lower-third vagina.**
IIA	Parametria is not involved.
IIB	Parametria is involved.
Stage III	**Invasion is to the pelvic wall or lower-third vagina.**
IIIA	Pelvic wall is not involved.
IIIB	Pelvic wall is involved; hydronephrosis of kidney
Stage IV	**Invasion is beyond the true pelvis or to bladder mucosa or rectum.**
IVA	Spread is to adjacent organs.
IVB	Spread is to adjacent organs.

FIGO = International Federation of Gynecology and Obstetrics

2. **Exam.** With advanced disease, a friable, bleeding cervical lesion or mass is seen.

3. **Diagnosis.** The definitive diagnosis can only be made by a cervical **biopsy.**

E. **Management** is based on staging, which is performed clinically.

1. Stage **IA1** is managed with a simple total hysterectomy.

2. Stage **IA2** is managed with a modified radical hysterectomy.

3. Stages **IB and II** are managed with either radical hysterectomy with bilateral lymph node dissection (for premenopausal women to preserve ovarian follicles) or radiation therapy (for postmenopausal women).

4. Stages **III and IV** are managed with radiation therapy.

Clinical Situation 24–1

Basic Case: A 38-year-old woman undergoes routine cervical Pap smear screening.

Patient Snapshot	Intervention	Clinical Pearls
The Pap smear report states **unsatisfactory for evaluation.**	Repeat the Pap smear in 6–12 weeks.	The screening test did not give usable information so it needs to be repeated.
The Pap smear report states **negative for CIN or malignancy** but evidence of trichomoniasis.	Only treat for trichomoniasis.	With CIN and malignancy ruled out, there is **no need to repeat** the Pap smear.
The Pap smear report shows **ASC-US.**	Any of the following: repeat Pap in 4–6 months, obtain HPV DNA-testing or colposcopic directed biopsies	Most ASC-US Pap smears are caused by benign HPV types that will frequently **spontaneously reverse** from immune system clearance of the virus. Conservative management without biopsy is appropriate.
The Pap smear report shows **ASC-H, LSIL, or HSIL.**	Colposcopic directed biopsies of punctuation, mosaicism, white epithelium, or abnormal vessels	Pap smear findings other than ASC-US may represent **persistent lesions** that could lead to cancer. Directed biopsy of abnormal epithelium is essential.
The Pap smear report shows **cancer.**	Colposcopic directed biopsies; biopsies of punctuation, mosaicism, white epithelium, or abnormal vessels	Biopsy areas of abnormal **vessels** that characterize invasive CA. It is imperative to know the **depth of invasion** through the basement membrane for **cancer staging.**

CIN = cervical intraepithelial neoplasia
ASC-US = atypical squamous cells of uncertain significance
ASC-H = ASC cannot exclude high-grade lesion

LSIL = low-grade squamous intraepithelial lesion
HSIL = high-grade squamous intraepithelial lesion
CA = cancer

Clinical Situation 24–2

Basic Case: A 38-year-old woman undergoes routine cervical Pap smear screening. The Pap smear is abnormal. Colposcopy and directed biopsies have been performed.

Patient Snapshot	Intervention	Clinical Pearls
The Pap smear shows **HSIL.** The colposcopy is **unsatisfactory** because the transformation zone is seen extending into the EC canal.	Perform an endocervical curettage (ECC). Also perform exocervical biopsies.	An ECC is necessary to screen for an unseen lesion in the EC canal. Cold knife cone is not needed if the ECC comes back **negative.**
The Pap smear shows **HSIL.** The colposcopy is **unsatisfactory** because a lesion is seen extending into the EC canal.	Perform a diagnostic excision procedure (cold knife cone). Also perform exocervical biopsies.	A deep cone biopsy is necessary to surgically excise the distal EC canal and any lesion within it.
The Pap smear showed **ASC-H or LSIL.** Colposcopy was **satisfactory.** Biopsies showed **CIN 1.**	Observe and follow-up without treatment using repeat Pap, colposcopy, or HPV DNA testing.	The majority of mild dysplasias undergo **spontaneous involution. Ablative** therapy (cryotherapy, laser) is also appropriate. Follow-up in 4–6 months.
The Pap smear showed **LSIL or HSIL.** Colposcopy was **satisfactory.** Biopsies showed **CIN 2 or 3.**	Perform **ablation** or **excision** (LEEP or cold cone) of the entire transformation zone.	Advanced CIN (2 or 3) lesions cannot be expected to spontaneously involute so they **must be removed** by ablation or excision. Follow-up to assess for recurrence.
Biopsies showed **CIN 3.** Primary therapy was **ablation** therapy. Follow-up biopsies showed **recurrent CIN 3.**	Perform **excision** procedure to remove the lesions.	Recurrent CIN after primary ablation therapy calls for excision therapy. **Do not repeat ablation.**
Biopsies showed **CIN 3.** Primary therapy was **excision** therapy. Follow-up biopsies showed **recurrent CIN 3.**	Consider **TVH or TAH.**	Hysterectomy is never acceptable for primary therapy for CIN 2, 3, but is **acceptable for recurrent CIN 2, 3.**
The Pap smear showed **HSIL.** The biopsies showed **CIN 2 or 3.**	Perform an ablative or excisional procedure of the entire T-zone.	Intraepithelial lesions (moderate dysplasia or worse) require **destruction** or **removal** of the epithelium.

CIN = cervical intraepithelial lesion
HPV DNA = human papilloma virus DNA
LSIL = low-grade squamous intraepithelial lesion
HSIL = high-grade squamous intraepithelial lesion

LEEP = loop electrosurgical excision procedure
TAH = total abdominal hysterectomy
TVH = total vaginal hysterectomy

Clinical Situation 24–3

Basic Case: A 43-year-old woman undergoes a routine cervical Pap smear screening. The Pap smear shows high-grade SIL, and an **ECC** report shows dysplastic cells.

Patient Snapshot	Intervention	Clinical Pearls
Colposcopy shows a **lesion extending into the endocervical canal.**	Perform deep cone biopsy.	A deep cone biopsy is necessary to surgically excise the distal endocervical canal and any lesion within it.
The cervical biopsy report shows **histologic changes less severe than expected** by Pap smear.	Perform shallow cone biopsy.	It must be assumed the site of the dysplastic Pap smear cells was not identified by colposcopy and biopsy. A wide but shallow cone biopsy, excising the entire T-zone, identifies the source of abnormal Pap smear cells.
The cervical biopsy shows **microinvasive squamous cell CA.**	Perform wide cone biopsy.	Wider cone biopsy excision ensures that areas next to the microinvasive CA are not frankly invasive cancer. Management of the two lesions is very different.
The cervical biopsy shows **adenocarcinoma in situ.**	Perform deep cone biopsy.	Adenocarcinoma usually arises within the endocervical canal. A deep cone biopsy is necessary to excise the distal endocervical canal surgically, making sure invasive cancer is not present.

CA = carcinoma   SIL = squamous epithelial lesion   T-zone = transition zone
ECC = endocervical curettage

Clinical Situation 24–4

Basic Case: A multiparous woman undergoes routine cervical Pap smear screening. The Pap smear is abnormal. Colposcopy and directed biopsies are performed.

Patient Snapshot	Intervention	Clinical Pearls
The patient is 35 years of age. Cervical biopsy shows invasive CA, **stage Ia1.**	Perform TAH or TVH.	With **minimal penetration** of the basement membrane by the tumor, the risk of metastasis is negligible.
The patient is 35 years of age. Cervical biopsy shows invasive CA, **stage Ia2.**	Perform modified radical hysterectomy.	With tumor **penetration < 5 mm,** risk of metastasis is more than stage **Ia1** but still not high.
The patient is 35 years of age. Cervical biopsy shows invasive CA, **stage Ib or II.**	Perform radical hysterectomy.	With **invasion > 5 mm,** wide surgical excision is needed because local metastasis has been confirmed. Ovarian function is preserved by surgical therapy in premenopausal women.
The patient is 60 years of age. Cervical biopsy shows invasive CA, **stage Ib or II.**	Recommend radiation therapy.	The 5-year survival rate after treatment with radiation therapy is equal to that after radical hysterectomy. Because loss of ovarian follicle function is not an issue in postmenopausal women, nonsurgical therapy is preferred.
The patient is 45 years of age. The cervical biopsy and pelvic exam are consistent with invasive CA, **stage III or IV.**	Recommend radiation therapy.	Stage III or IV cervical CA is treated by radiation therapy regardless of patient age.
The patient is 35 years of age and **pregnant.** Biopsy shows invasive cervical cancer.	Manage based on cancer staging and gestational age.	Therapy type is based on tumor stage. If gestational age at diagnosis is prior to viability, ignore the pregnancy and start treatment. If the fetus is viable or close to it, temporary treatment deferral may be appropriate.

CA = carcinoma   TAH = total abdominal hysterectomy   TVH = total vaginal hysterectomy

25

Vulvar Neoplasia and Cancer

I. VULVAR DYSTROPHY

A. Definition. Vulvar dystrophy represents a spectrum of hyperplastic and/or atrophic benign lesions that may have clinical findings similar to those of vulvar carcinoma.

B. Clinical findings

   1. Symptoms. Itching is the *most common* complaint. Dysuria, dyspareunia, and vulvodynia also occur.

   2. Examination
      a. Squamous hyperplasia. White, firm, cartilaginous lesions are evident.
      b. Lichen sclerosis. A thin, bluish, parchment-like appearance with labial fusion is present. Scarring and contracture may be seen.

   3. Diagnosis. The basis of diagnosis is **vulvar biopsy (Figure 25–1).**

C. Management

   1. Squamous hyperplasia. Treatment involves topical fluorinated corticosteroids.

   2. Lichen sclerosis. Treatment involves topical clobestasol, a high potency steroid.

II. VULVAR INTRAEPITHELIAL NEOPLASIA (VIN)

A. Definition. VIN refers to vulvar cellular atypia present only **within the epithelium** without penetrating the basement membrane.

B. Epidemiology

   1. Risk factors include obesity; chronic hypertension; and infection with **human papilloma virus (HPV), types 16 and 18.**

   2. VIN may be found **in association with CIN.**

C. Clinical findings

   1. Symptoms. Itching or irritation is common, but many patients are asymptomatic.

   2. Examination. Lesions may appear white, red, or pigmented; they are usually discrete and often multifocal.

D. Diagnosis. Vulvar biopsy provides the diagnosis.

E. Management. Involved epithelial areas should be **surgically excised** or **vaporized with a laser.**

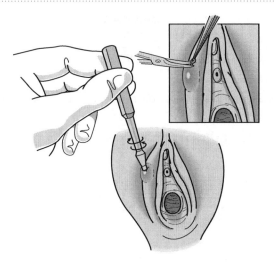

Figure 25–1. Punch biopsy of vulvar lesion.

III. VULVAR CANCER

A. Epidemiology

  1. Prevalence. Vulvar cancer is the **fourth most common gynecologic malignancy (5%),** with **average age at diagnosis of 65 years.**

  2. **Risk factors** include obesity; chronic hypertension; and infection with **HPV, types 16 and 18.**

  3. No formal **screening** test exists. Visually identified vulvar lesions are biopsied.

B. Pathophysiology

  1. **Multifocal areas** of squamous epithelium dysplasia may arise on the **vulva** and contiguous areas such as the **anus** and **clitoris.** The *most common* **tumor** (90%) is of the squamous or epidermoid type. Melanoma is much less common.

  2. **Invasive cancer** is diagnosed when the full-thickness changes of carcinoma in situ (CIS) break **through the basement membrane. Progression** to invasive carcinoma is less frequent in the vulva than with the cervix.

  3. Route of spread
    a. The *most common* **primary spread** occurs by **direct extension.**
    b. **Lymphatic spread** occurs from the superficial to the deep inguinal nodes.

C. Clinical findings

  1. **Symptoms.** Early disease may be **asymptomatic,** but **itching** is the *most common* **symptom.**

  2. **Examination.** An inflamed or bleeding vulvar lesion or mass is present.

  3. **Diagnosis.** Definitive diagnosis can be made only by vulvar **biopsy.**

D. **Staging (Table 25–1).** Note that staging is performed **surgically.**

E. **Management.** Basic treatment is **radical vulvectomy** with bilateral **inguinal lymph node dissection.** Radiation therapy and chemotherapy are only adjunctive.

Table 25–1
Surgical Staging of Vulvar Carcinoma

FIGO Stage	Description
Stage 0	Carcinoma-in-situ; confined to the epithelium
Stage I	Tumor confined to vulva; ≤ 2 cm in size; negative inguinal nodes
Stage II	Tumor confined to vulva; > 2 cm in size; negative inguinal nodes
Stage III	Tumor of any size with spread to lower urethra, vagina, or anus; unilateral inguinal nodes positive
Stage IVa	Tumor invasion of upper urethra, mucosa of bladder/rectum, pelvic bone; bilateral inguinal nodes positive
Stage IVb	Any distant metastasis, including pelvic nodes

FIGO = International Federation of Gynecology and Obstetrics

Clinical Situation 25–1

Basic Case: A 65-year-old woman comes to the office concerned about a vulvar lesion that she states has caused itching for 6 months.

Patient Snapshot	Intervention	Clinical Pearls
On exam you find a 6- × 10-mm lesion on her left labia majora.	Perform vulvar biopsy.	**Biopsy is imperative.** It is not possible to differentiate benign from malignant lesions by visual inspection.
➥ **Scenario 1** Diagnosis on biopsy is **squamous hyperplasia.**	Administer fluorinated corticosteroid cream.	The lesions are white in color and firm and cartilaginous to the touch because of thickened keratin.
➥ **Scenario 2** Diagnosis on biopsy is **lichen sclerosis.**	Administer clobestasol cream.	The lesions are bluish-white and thin and parchment-like to the touch because of epithelial thinning.
➥ **Scenario 3** Diagnosis on biopsy is **moderate dysplasia.**	Perform surgical excision.	This is an intraepithelial premalignant condition that should be removed.
➥ **Scenario 4** Diagnosis on biopsy is **carcinoma-in-situ,** or stage 0 vulvar CA.	Perform skinning vulvectomy or laser ablation.	This represents full-thickness loss of cellular polarity, but the basement membrane is intact.
➥ **Scenario 5** Diagnosis on biopsy is **invasive squamous cell CA.**	Perform radical vulvectomy and bilateral lymph node dissection.	Staging for vulvar CA is surgical. This requires radical surgery for determining if inguinal lymph nodes are involved.

CA = carcinoma

26

Breast Disease

I. **BENIGN BREAST DISEASE.** Common benign breast changes include generalized changes, breast lumps, nipple discharge, and infection.

   A. **Fibrocystic changes.** This is the *most common* **benign breast condition.** This generalized **painful** condition occurs most often in women 20 to 50 years old and are an exaggerated response to the cyclic levels of ovarian hormones.

   1. Examination shows the cysts occur bilaterally and may vary in size from nonpalpable to many cm.

   2. Diagnosis is confirmed by sonogram showing fluid filled cysts.

   3. Management of gross cysts is fine-needle aspiration. Medical management varies from reducing caffeine intake and taking oral vitamin E to suppression of cyclic hormonal changes with oral contraceptives, bromocriptine, and tamoxifen.

   B. **Fibroadenomas.** These are the *most common* **benign breast tumors in young women.** These **painless,** usually unilateral breast lumps occur more often in Black than White women. Etiology is unknown.

   1. Examination reveals a mobile, firm, smooth, rubbery lump with size ranging up to 5 cm or more.

   2. Diagnosis is confirmed by sonogram showing a solid, smooth, uniform solid breast mass. Fine-needle aspiration shows a typical appearance.

   3. Management may be conservative in stable, smaller masses in young women. Larger masses may best be removed by excisional biopsy.

   C. **Fat necrosis.** This **painful** condition occurs typically in obese women with pendulous breasts and is the result of local tissue trauma.

   1. Examination demonstrates a firm, tender, indurated, ill-defined breast mass of varying size. Skin or nipple retraction may be noted

   2. Diagnosis requires fine-needle aspiration or open biopsy. Mammography cannot distinguish benign from malignant changes.

   3. Management is conservative after the diagnosis is confirmed.

   D. **Sclerosing adenosis.** This **painful** condition is the result of excessive growth of tissues in the breast's lobules and may vary with the menstrual cycle.

   1. Examination demonstrates a firm, tender, indurated, ill-defined breast mass of varying size. Skin or nipple retraction may be noted.

2. **Diagnosis** requires fine-needle aspiration or open biopsy. Mammography may show calcifications indistinguishable from carcinoma.

3. **Management** is conservative after the diagnosis is confirmed.

E. **Intraductal papilloma.** This condition is the ***most common* benign cause of bloody nipple discharge.** It occurs most often in women between the ages of 30 and 50 years. The bleeding arises from small, benign tumors within the breast milk duct.

1. **Examination** reveals unilateral bloody nipple discharge often without a palpable mass.

2. **Diagnosis** requires fine-needle aspiration or open biopsy. Mammographic and sonographic findings are not definitive.

3. **Management** is conservative after the diagnosis is confirmed.

F. **Duct ectasia.** This painless condition results from inflammatory dilation of the mammary ducts and occurs most often in peri and postmenopausal women.

1. **Examination** reveals sticky, greenish-black or bloody nipple discharge, often bilateral, with or without a palpable mass.

2. **Diagnosis** requires open biopsy. Mammography is obtained to rule out carcinoma but is not diagnostic.

3. **Management** is conservative after the diagnosis is confirmed.

G. **Cystosarcoma phyllodes.** This rare, **nontender,** unilateral lesion is the ***most common* nonepithelial neoplasm of the breast.** It usually occurs in women in their 40s. It often enlarges rapidly and is usually benign but may be malignant. This large, bulky lesion has similarities to fibroadenomas.

1. **Examination** reveals a firm, smooth, mobile breast mass 5 cm or larger in size usually removed from the nipple area.

2. **Diagnosis** requires excision with a wide margin to minimize recurrence. Mammography is obtained to rule out carcinoma but is not diagnostic.

3. **Management** is close follow-up to rule out local recurrence or malignancy.

II. **MALIGNANT BREAST DISEASE.** Breast cancer is the ***most common* female malignancy** with 1 in 9 lifetime risk.

A. **Risk factors.** Most women who develop breast cancer have no identifiable risk factors.

1. **Genetics.** Family history with a first degree relative increases risk 2- to 3-fold. **BRAC1 and 2 gene carriers** have up to 50% risk of breast cancer.

2. **Prolonged unopposed estrogen** is the probable mediating factor with increased risk from: early menarche, late menopause, nulliparity, late age at first pregnancy, age over 40 years.

3. **Hyperplasia or cellular atypia** found on biopsy with fibrocystic disease increases risk 2- to 4-fold.

4. **Others.** High dietary fat intake, history of breast irradiation, obesity

B. **Types**

1. **Infiltrating ductal.** This is the ***most common* breast malignancy** accounting for 80% of all breast cancers. This mostly unilateral lesion probably begins as ductal carcinoma in situ **(DCIS),** which then invades the basement membrane becoming invasive ductal carcinoma. With increasing size and fibrotic tissue response the tumor becomes palpable as a stony hard mass.

2. **Infiltrating lobular.** These tumors account for 10% of all breast cancers. They orig-inate in the breast lobules and are frequently bilateral. They probably begin as lob-ular carcinoma in situ (LCIS) which then invades the basement membrane to become invasive cancer. Prognosis of lobular invasive cancer is better than ductal carcinoma.

3. **Inflammatory.** Although this is an uncommon breast cancer, it is rapidly growing with early metastasis potential. The tumor blocks the lymphatic vessels in the breast skin resulting in redness, swelling and warmth on examination. The ede-matous skin may appear pitted, like the skin of an orange (called *peau d'orange*).

4. **Paget's disease.** This is an uncommon breast cancer. The most common sign is a pruritic, red, scaly rash involving the nipple, which may spread to the areola. The nipple may be inverted (pulled in) and there may also be some discharge. The symptoms of Paget's disease can look like other skin conditions such as eczema or psoriasis. Prognosis of Paget's disease is better than ductal carcinoma.

C. Detection and diagnosis

1. **Breast exam.** The majority of breast masses are discovered by patients during self-examination. Breast self-exam **(BSE)** should be explained to all women beginning in their 20s. They should be told about the benefits and limitations of BSE. Since randomized trials have not demonstrated a benefit, women can elect to either per-form or not perform regular BSE. BSEs are not a substitute for regular clinical breast exams **(CBE)** by a health professional. Women in their 20s and 30s should have CBE as part of a routine physical, at least every three years. At 40 years of age and thereafter, CBE should be done annually.

2. **Ultrasound.** The most important use of this imaging modality is to differentiate solid from cystic masses. It should not be used as a screening test for subclinical dis-ease since small lesions and microcalcifications are not visualized.

3. **Mammography.** This is the most accurate conventional method of detecting non-palpable breast carcinoma. It is more sensitive in older rather than younger women. It can detect microcalcifications and masses below the threshold of pal-pation. Current ACS recommendations are: women at average risk for breast can-cer should start mammographic screening at age 40 years with repeat exams every 1–2 years; women with genetic risk factors should start between ages 25 to 35 years.

4. **Fine-needle aspiration (FNA).** This outpatient procedure is performed without anesthetic. If aspiration of a cystic mass yields clear fluid, no further testing is needed. Bloody or turbid fluid should be sent for cytology and open biopsy con-sidered. With solid lesions several passes are made through the mass with contin-uous suction from the syringe. The cellular specimen within the needle is placed on a slide and fixed for analysis. If the physical exam, imaging findings, and cy-tology are benign, the mass can be safely followed. Otherwise open biopsy is needed.

5. **Open biopsy.** This outpatient procedure, performed under local anesthesia, yields the definitive diagnosis for breast disease. Indications include: bloody nipple dis-charge, persistent mass after FNA, suspicious mammography, nipple retraction, sus-picious skin changes.

6. **Stereotactic core-needle biopsy (CNB).** CNB can be performed on most nonpal-pable, suspicious abnormalities seen on high-quality mammography. The breast biopsy path is stereotactically imaged from two slightly angled directions to help guide the needle. Small samples of tissue are then removed from the breast using a hollow core needle or vacuum-assisted biopsy device.

7. **Sentinel node biopsy.** By injecting the primary tumor with radioactive tracer, the surgeon can identify the first set of regional lymph nodes that receive lymphatic drainage from the tumor. Axillary node dissection can be omitted if the sentinel nodes are negative.

D. Treatment options are selected based on tumor staging. **Primary** therapy is used to remove or destroy **identified** tumor and surrounding tissue. **Adjuvant** therapy is used to kill distant spread of **undetected** cancer cells.

1. **Surgery.** Breast-saving **lumpectomy** removes the tumor and a rim of normal tissues surrounding it. This is the treatment of choice in early-stage breast cancer (along with radiation therapy) for unilateral small tumors (< 4 cm size). Breast-removing surgery includes: **simple mastectomy** (removal of only the breast) may be performed for widespread DCIS or LCIS, and **modified radical mastectomy** (removal of the breast and axillary nodes) may be performed for larger tumors followed by immediate breast reconstructive surgery. **Radical mastectomy** (removal of the breast, axillary nodes, and the chest muscles under the breast) is almost never performed today because it does not improve survival.

2. **Radiation therapy (RT).** This modality is always included as **primary** therapy after breast conserving surgery. It is started a month after surgery and continued for six weeks. RT is used as **adjuvant** therapy if given before or after breast-removing mastectomy to destroy remaining cancer cells or shrink tumors with advanced breast cancer.

3. **Hormone therapy.** The goal of hormone therapy is to prevent breast cancer cells from receiving stimulation from estrogen. This modality is useful if the tumor is estrogen or progesterone receptor positive. Receptor negative tumors tend to be more aggressive than hormone positive ones and do not respond to hormone therapy. Estrogen deprivation can be achieved either through destruction/removal of ovaries or administration of medications. **Tamoxifen** (Nolvadex), a selective estrogen receptor modulator **(SERM),** may be used prophylactically with early stage breast cancer as well therapeutically with advanced or recurrent cancer. **Aromatase inhibitors** (anastrozole [Arimidex], letrozole [Femara]) are new hormone therapy drugs.

4. **Chemotherapy.** The goal of systemic chemotherapy is to destroy breast cancer cells outside the surgical margins. Most patients receiving hormone therapy also are given chemotherapy. Multiple agent cytotoxic chemotherapy is used in most women with lymph node metastases or with primary breast cancers larger than 1 cm in diameter (both node-negative and node-positive). For women with node-negative cancers less than 1 cm in diameter, the decision to consider chemotherapy should be individualized. Agents used include: doxorubicin (Adriamycin) (A), cyclophosphamide (C), vincristine (V), as well as methotrexate (M).

Appendix A

What Is the Most Common . . .?

Note: The first column describes the feature referred to as "*most common*" in the text, which is the one that completes the question given in the table title, the second column gives the answer, and the third column lists the text reference telling where the answer can be found.

Most Common Feature in Question	*Most Common* Answer	Text Reference
Fundal height at 12 weeks' gestation	At symphysis pubis	Chapter 1 VII D 1
Fundal height at 16 weeks' gestation	Midway between pubis and umbilicus	Chapter 1 VII D 2
Fundal height at 20 weeks' gestation	At umbilicus	Chapter 1 VII D 3
Cause of apparent discrepant fundal size	Measurement error or dating error	Chapter 1 VIII B
Cause of symmetric IUGR	Decreased fetal growth potential	Chapter 1 VIII D 1
Cause of asymmetric IUGR	Inadequate nutritional substrate availability	Chapter 1 VIII D 2
Cause of first-trimester loss	Aneuploidy (abnormal embryo karyotype)	Chapter 2 I B
Type of fetal aneuploidy	Autosomal trisomy	Chapter 2 I B
Type of single aneuploidy	Monosomy X (Turner syndrome)	Chapter 2 I B
Cause of second-trimester loss	Uterine anomalies	Chapter 2 I C
Clinical findings with uterine duplication	Preterm cervical dilation and labor with painful contractions	Chapter 2 I C 1 a
Clinical finding with incompetent cervix	Preterm painless cervical dilation	Chapter 2 I C 1 c
Method of diagnosing uterine anomalies	Hysterosalpingogram	Chapter 2 I C 2 a
Management of thin uterine septum	Hysteroscopic resection	Chapter 2 I C 3 a
Management of incompetent cervix	Cervical cerclage	Chapter 2 I C 3 b
Evidence of early fetal demise	Lack of fundal growth	Chapter 2 II A 1 a
Evidence of later fetal demise	Absence of fetal movements	Chapter 2 II A 1 b
Confirmation of fetal demise	Absence of cardiac motion on sonography	Chapter 2 II A 2
Cause of fetal demise	Idiopathic; no cause identified	Chapter 2 II B 1
Cause of DIC with prolonged fetal demise	Release of fetal tissue thromboplastin into the maternal circulation	Chapter 2 II C 1
Type of hydatidiform mole	Complete mole	Chapter 2 III A 1 a
Karyotype of complete mole	Normal, diploidy (46, XX)	Chapter 2 III A 1 a

Note: The first column describes the feature referred to as "*most common*" in the text, which is the one that completes the question given in the table title, the second column gives the answer, and the third column lists the text reference telling where the answer can be found.

Most Common Feature in Question	*Most Common* Answer	Text Reference
Karyotype of incomplete mole	Abnormal, triploidy (69,XXY)	Chapter 2 III A 1 b
Site of metastasis with good prognosis malignant GTD	Lung or pelvis	Chapter 2 III A 2 a
Site of metastasis with poor prognosis malignant GTD	Brain or liver	Chapter 2 III A 2 b
Clinical finding with GTD	Bleeding < 16 weeks' gestation	Chapter 2 III B 1
Cause of preeclampsia < 20 weeks' gestation	GTD	Chapter 2 III B 1
Management of GTD	Suction D&C and follow serial β-hCG titers	Chapter 2 III C 1, 3, 5
Chemotherapy for GTD	Methotrexate and actinomycin D	Chapter 2 III C 6
Location of ectopic pregnancy	Distal oviduct	Chapter 2 IV A 2
Pathophysiology for ectopic pregnancy	Intratubal adhesions	Chapter 2 IV A 3
Risk factor for ectopic pregnancy	Previous salpingitis	Chapter 2 IV A 3 a
Symptom triad for ectopic pregnancy	Amenorrhea, vaginal bleeding, abdominal pain	Chapter 2 IV B 1
Management of ectopic pregnancy ≤ 7 weeks' gestation	IV methotrexate	Clinical Situation 2-5
Management of ectopic pregnancy > 7 weeks' gestation	Laparoscopy	Clinical Situation 2-5
Cause of abnormal high or low MS-AFP	Pregnancy dating error	Chapter 3 I B 1 a
Follow-up for abnormal MS-AFP	Sonogram to identify if dating error	Chapter 3 I B 1 a; Clinical Situation 3-1
Follow-up for high MS-AFP after sonogram confirms dates	Amniocentesis for AF-AFP level and acetyl-cholinesterase	Clinical Situation 3-1
Gestational age for sonography fetal anomaly screening	18–20 weeks' gestation	Chapter 3 I B 1 c
Follow-up for low MS-AFP after sonogram confirms dates	Amniocentesis for karyotype to rule out aneuploidy	Chapter 3 I B 2 b; Clinical Situation 3-1
Cause of fetal anomalies	Polygenic/multifactorial (65%)	Chapter 3 I C 1
Kind of single-gene disorder associated with gross anatomic lesions	Autosomal dominant	Chapter 3 I C 2 a
Kind of single-gene disorder associated with biochemical disorders	Autosomal recessive	Chapter 3 I C 2 b
Kind of single-gene disorder transmitted to offspring on X chromosome	Sex-linked recessive	Chapter 3 I C 2 c
Specific autosomal trisomy	Trisomy 21, Down syndrome	Chapter 3 I C 3
Indications for antenatal fetal testing	DM and postdates pregnancy	Chapter 3 II A 2
Antenatal fetal testing method	NST	Chapter 3 II B 2
Explanation for reactive NST	Healthy fetus that is moving	Chapter 3 II B 2
Follow-up for reactive NST	Repeat test weekly or biweekly	Chapter 3 II B 2 a

Note: The first column describes the feature referred to as "*most common*" in the text, which is the one that completes the question given in the table title, the second column gives the answer, and the third column lists the text reference telling where the answer can be found.

Most Common Feature in Question	*Most Common* Answer	Text Reference
Explanation for nonreactive NST	Healthy fetus that may be asleep, immature, or sedated	Chapter 3 II B 2 b
Follow-up for nonreactive NST	VAS	Chapter 3 II B 2 b (1)
Explanation for negative CST	Adequate intervillous blood flow in the presence of 3 UCs in 10 minutes	Chapter 3 II B 3 a; Figure 3-2
Follow-up for negative CST	Repeat test weekly	Chapter 3 II B 3 a
Explanation for positive CST combined with nonreactive NST	Compromised fetus	Chapter 3 II B 3 b
Follow-up for positive CST with nonreactive NST	Prompt delivery	Chapter 3 II B 3 b
Follow-up for BPP score of 8 or 10	Repeat test weekly	Chapter 3 II B 4 b (1)
Follow-up for BPP score of 4 or 6	Prompt delivery if ≥ 36 weeks; otherwise repeat in 24 hours	Chapter 3 II B 4 b (2)
Follow-up for BPP score of 0 or 2	Prompt delivery	Chapter 3 II B 4 b (3)
Outcome with nonreassuring EFM strip	Healthy infant with good Apgar scores	Chapter 3 III C
Anatomic abnormality in presence of true elevation of MS-AFP	Open NTD	Table 3-1
Teratogenic effect of alcohol	Midfacial hypoplasia	Table 3-2
Teratogenic effect of streptomycin	VIII nerve damage	Table 3-2
Follow-up with accelerations on intrapartum EFM	Conservative management	Clinical Situation 3-4
Follow-up with early decelerations on intrapartum EFM	Conservative management	Clinical Situation 3-4
Follow-up with variable decelerations on intrapartum EFM	Conservative management if mild or moderate; prompt delivery if severe	Clinical Situation 3-4
Follow-up with late decelerations on intrapartum EFM	Prompt delivery if severe	Clinical Situation 3-4
Follow-up fetal scalp pH ≥ 7.20	Conservative management	Clinical Situation 3-4
Follow-up fetal scalp pH < 7.20	Prompt delivery	Clinical Situation 3-4
Diagnostic modality for multiple gestation	Obstetric sonogram	Chapter 4 II B
Type of zygosity of twins	Dizygous	Table 4-1
Type of chorionicity of twins	Dichorionic	Table 4-1
Type of amnionicity of twins	Diamniotic	Table 4-1
Presentation of twins in labor	Cephalic-cephalic	Chapter 4 VI A 1
Route of delivery with cephalic-cephalic twins	Vaginal delivery	Chapter 4 VI A 1
Route of delivery with breech-cephalic twins	Cesarean section	Chapter 4 VI A 3
Cause of painless third-trimester bleeding	Placenta previa	Chapter 5 III A
Cause of third-trimester bleeding	Abruptio placentae	Chapter 5 IV A
Cause of painful third-trimester bleeding	Abruptio placentae	Chapter 5 IV A
Obstetric cause of DIC	Abruptio placentae	Chapter 5 IV A
Specific Rh antigen causing isoimmunization	D antigen	Chapter 6 I B

Note: The first column describes the feature referred to as "*most common*" in the text, which is the one that completes the question given in the table title, the second column gives the answer, and the third column lists the text reference telling where the answer can be found.

Most Common Feature in Question	*Most Common* Answer	Text Reference
Indication for RhoGAM in pregnancy	Route 28-week antepartum prophylaxis	Chapter 6 III A 2
Clinical triad with preeclampsia	Hypertension, proteinuria, edema	Chapter 7 II A
Type of hypertensive disorder of pregnancy	Mild preeclampsia	Chapter 7 II B 1
Risk factor for preeclampsia	Nulliparity	Chapter 7 III A
Type of glucose intolerance in pregnancy	GDM	Chapter 8 I B 1 a
Mechanism of glucose intolerance in GDM	Anti-insulin effect of hPL	Chapter 8 I B 1 a
Complication of diabetes resulting in polyhydramnios	Poor glucose control	Chapter 8 II A 1 a
Pathophysiology of fetal anomalies in diabetic pregnancies	Poor glucose control during embryogenesis	Chapter 8 II B 1 a
Type of fetal anomalies in diabetic pregnancies	NTDs and cardiac anomalies	Chapter 8 II B 1 b
Type of fetal growth disorder in diabetic fetuses	Macrosomia	Chapter 8 II B 2 a
Screening test for GDM	1-hr 50-g OGTT	Chapter 8 IV B
Type of anemia in pregnancy	Iron deficiency anemia	Chapter 9 I B 1
Etiology of heart disease in pregnancy	Acquired heart disease	Chapter 9 II D 1
Acquired heart disease lesion found in pregnant women	Mitral stenosis	Chapter 9 II D 1 a
Congenital heart disease lesion found in pregnant women	ASD or VSD	Chapter 9 II D 2 a
Cyanotic heart disease lesion found in pregnant women	Tetralogy of Fallot	Chapter 9 II D 2 b
Source of UTIs in women	Ascending from vagina or rectum	Chapter 9 III B
Causal organism of UTIs in women	*Escherichia coli*	Chapter 9 III B
Type of UTI in pregnancy	Asymptomatic bacteriuria	Chapter 9 III C 1
Serious medical complication in pregnancy	Acute pyelonephritis	Chapter 9 III C 3
Anatomic site of venous thrombosis in pregnancy	Pelvic or lower extremity veins	Chapter 9 IV D
Type of pruritic dermatosis in pregnancy	PUPPP syndrome	Chapter 9 IV F
Fetal lie in utero	Longitudinal lie	Chapter 10 I A 1
Fetal presentation in utero	Cephalic presentation	Chapter 10 I A 2
Fetal position in utero	Occiput anterior position	Chapter 10 I A 3
Fetal attitude in utero	Vertex presentation	Chapter 10 I A 4
Classification of forceps used	Outlet forceps	Chapter 10 III A 1 a
Indication for primary cesarean section	Cephalopelvic disproportion	Chapter 10 III B 1 a
Uterine incision for cesarean section	Low segment transverse	Chapter 10 III B 2 a
Neonatal effect of maternal intra-partum narcotics	Neonatal respiratory depression	Table 10-3
Fetal effect of maternal intrapartum paracervical block	Fetal bradycardia	Table 10-3
Maternal vascular effect of epidural block	Maternal hypotension	Table 10-3

Note: The first column describes the feature referred to as "*most common*" in the text, which is the one that completes the question given in the table title, the second column gives the answer, and the third column lists the text reference telling where the answer can be found.

Most Common Feature in Question	*Most Common* Answer	Text Reference
Diagnosis leading to neonatal ICU admissions	PROM	Chapter 11 I A 2
Risk factor for PROM	Ascending infection from lower gential tract	Chapter 11 I C 1
Morbidity in premature infants	RDS	Chapter 11 I D 2 a
Cause of neonatal deaths in United States	Preterm delivery	Chapter 11 II A 2
Obstetric history risk factor associated with preterm birth	Previous preterm delivery	Chapter 11 I B 2
Current pregnancy risk factor associated with preterm birth	Uterine anomaly	Chapter 11 II B 3
Tocolytic agent causing maternal respiratory depression	Magnesium sulfate	Chapter 11 II F 1 b
Tocolytic agent causing maternal hypokalemia	β-adrenergic agonists (e.g., terbutaline, ritodrine)	Chapter 11 II F 2 b
Tocolytic agent causing oligohydramnios	Prostaglandin synthetase inhibitors (e.g., indomethacin)	Chapter 11 II F 3 b
Tocolytic agent causing maternal myocardial depression	Calcium channel blockers (e.g., nifedipine)	Chapter 11 II F 4 b
Neonatal outcome of postdates pregnancy	Macrosomia syndrome	Chapter 11 III B 1
Length of anovulation with lactation	3 months	Chapter 12 I C
Cause of postpartum hemorrhage	Uterine atony	Chapter 12 II B 1
Risk factors for uterine atony	Rapid or protracted labor	Chapter 12 II B 1
Risk factor for genital laceration	Uncontrolled vaginal delivery	Chapter 12 II B 2
Risk factor for retained placenta	Noncontracted uterus	Chapter 12 II B 3
Risk factor for uterine inversion	Myometrial weakness	Chapter 12 II B 5
Cause of postpartum fever	Endometritis	Chapter 12 III D
Cause of genital ulcer disease	Herpes simplex	Chapter 13 I A 1
Classic lesion of primary syphilis	Painless chancre	Chapter 13 II A 2 a
Classic lesion of secondary syphilis	Condyloma lata	Chapter 13 II A 2 b
Classic lesion of tertiary syphilis	Gummas	Chapter 13 II A 2 d
Classic clinical sign of LGV	"Groove sign," double genitocrural fold	Chapter 13 II B 3
Type of STD overall	HPV	Chapter 13 III A 1
Type of viral STD	HPV	Chapter 13 III A 1
Cause of mucopurulent cervicitis	*Chlamydia trachomatis*	Chapter 13 III B 1
Neonatal manifestation of chlamydia	Inclusion conjunctivitis	Chapter 13 III B 1 a
Risk factor for female chlamydia	Sexual activity at age < 20 years	Chapter 13 III B 1 c
Antigen marker used for HBV screening	HBsAg	Chapter 13 III D 4
Antigen marker to predict infectivity	HBeAg	Chapter 13 III D 4
Screening test for HIV	ELISA	Chapter 13 III E 4 a
Diagnostic entity causing PID	Acute salpingo-oophoritis	Chapter 14 I
Type of bacterial STD	*Chlamydia trachomatis*	Chapter 14 I A 1
Secondary bacterial invaders with TOAs	Anaerobic bacteria (e.g., *Bacteroides* sp.)	Chapter 14 III D
Dominant vaginal microflora	Lactobacillus	Chapter 15 I A 3
Cause of abnormal vaginal discharge in United States	BV	Chapter 15 II

Note: The first column describes the feature referred to as "*most common*" in the text, which is the one that completes the question given in the table title, the second column gives the answer, and the third column lists the text reference telling where the answer can be found.

Most Common Feature in Question	*Most Common* Answer	Text Reference
Vaginal organisms in BV	Anaerobic bacteria	Chapter 15 II A
Candida species in yeast vaginitis	*Candida albicans*	Chapter 15 III
Cause of abnormal vaginal discharge worldwide	Trichomonas vaginitis	Chapter 15 IV
Cause of amenorrhea with low gonadotropins	Hypothalamic-pituitary abnormalities	Chapter 16 I B 1
Cause of amenorrhea with high gonadotropins	Ovarian follicular failure	Chapter 16 I B 2
Cause of amenorrhea with normal gonadotropins	Anovulation	Chapter 16 I B 3
Cause of primary amenorrhea overall	Gonadal dysgenesis	Chapter 16 II A 2 a
Cause of primary amenorrhea with breasts absent, uterus present	Gonadal dysgenesis	Chapter 16 II A 2 a
Cause of primary amenorrhea with breast present, uterus absent	Müllerian agenesis	Chapter 16 II B 1 a
Cause of secondary amenorrhea overall	Pregnancy	Chapter 16 III A
Cause of positive PCT	Anovulation	Chapter 16 III B 1
Cause of a positive EPCT	Lack of estrogen	Chapter 16 III C 1
Cause of a negative EPCT	Outflow tract obstruction	Chapter 16 III C 2
Cause of unpredictable, irregular, upper genital tract bleeding	Anovulation	Chapter 17 I B 1 a, b
Cause of abnormal bleeding between regular cycles	Uterine structural or anatomic lesions (e.g., endometrial polyps or submucous leiomyomas)	Chapter 17 I B 2 b
Cause of abnormal bleeding in reproductive years	Pregnancy	Chapter 17 I D 1
Correctable causes of anovulation	Pituitary prolactinoma or hypothyroidism	Chapter 17 I E 1 b (1)
Cause of primary dysmenorrhea	Prostaglandin-mediated uterine ischemia caused by progesterone withdrawal	Chapter 17 II A 2
Location of endometriosis lesions	Ovary	Chapter 17 III A
Pelvic examination findings in endometriosis	Retroverted uterus with uterosacral ligament nodularity	Chapter 17 III C
Successful treatment for PMS	SSRIs	Chapter 17 IV D 1
Initial pubertal change in girls	Thelarche (breast development)	Chapter 18 I B 3
Cause of true or central precocious puberty	Idiopathic (unexplained premature activation of a normal HPO axis)	Chapter 18 I C 1 a
Long-term effect of precocious puberty	Short stature	Chapter 18 I E 1
Mean age at menopause	51 years	Chapter 18 II A 1
Cause of menopause	Loss of functional ovarian follicles	Chapter 18 II B
Type of bone decreased in osteoporosis	Trabecular bone	Chapter 18 II D 1
Fracture site in osteoporosis	Vertebral body	Chapter 18 II D 1 c

Note: The first column describes the feature referred to as "***most common***" in the text, which is the one that completes the question given in the table title, the second column gives the answer, and the third column lists the text reference telling where the answer can be found.

Most Common Feature in Question	*Most Common* Answer	Text Reference
Cause of death in women	Cardiovascular disease	Chapter 18 II D 2
Effect of menopause on lipid profiles	Increased LDL and decreased HDL	Chapter 18 II D 2 a
Occurrence of uterine perforation by IUD	At time of insertion	Chapter 19 I E 5 a
Reversible contraceptive in United States	Estrogen–progestin contraceptive pills	Chapter 19 I F 1 a
Form of pregnancy prevention in United States	Female tubal sterilization	Chapter 19 II A 1
Objective criteria of vasectomy success	Azoospermia	Chapter 19 II A 2
Female cause of infertility	Anovulation	Chapter 19 III B 1
Pharmacologic treatment for anovulation	Clomiphene citrate	Chapter 19 III B 1 c (2)
Method of diagnosing fallopian tubal disease	HSG	Chapter 19 III B 2 b (1)
Male cause of infertility	Abnormal semen analysis	Chapter 19 III B 3
Abortion method type in United States	Suction D&C	Chapter 19 IV B 1
Cause of female incontinence overall	Genuine stress incontinence	Chapter 20 II C 1
Cause of incontinence with loss of bladder neck support	Genuine stress incontinence	Chapter 20 II C 1 a
Cause of incontinence with involuntary detrusor contractions	Hypertonic, motor urge incontinence	Chapter 20 II C 2 a (1)
Cause of incontinence with high bladder residual volumes	Hypotonic, overflow incontinence	Chapter 20 II C 3 a (2)
Cause of incontinence with history of radical pelvic surgery	Bypass incontinence with urinary tract fistula	Chapter 20 II C 4
Cause of an enlarged uterus in reproductive years	Pregnancy	Chapter 21 I
Type of uterine tumor	Leiomyoma	Chapter 21 II
Racial group predisposed to uterine leiomyomas	Black women	Chapter 21 II
Time of occurrence of increase in size of uterine leiomyomas	Pregnancy	Chapter 21 II A 3
Anatomic site of uterine leiomyomas associated with abnormal bleeding	Submucous leiomyomas	Chapter 21 II C 1
Diagnosis with nonpregnant, non-tender, enlarged, firm, asymmetrical uterus	Uterine leiomyomas	Chapter 21 II D
Diagnosis with nonpregnant, tender, enlarged, soft, symmetrical uterus	Uterine adenomyosis	Chapter 21 III C
Pathophysiology of endometrial hyperplasia	Unopposed estrogen stimulation	Chapter 22 I B
Premalignant histology of endometrial hyperplasia	Complex hyperplasia with atypia	Chapter 22 I B 3
Type of gynecologic malignancy	Endometrial carcinoma	Chapter 22 II A 1
Tumor type of endometrial carcinoma	Endometrial adenocarcinoma	Chapter 22 II A 1
Primary route of spread of endometrial carcinoma	Direct extension to the endometrium and cervix	Chapter 22 II B
Symptom of endometrial carcinoma	Postmenopausal bleeding	Chapter 22 II C 1

Note: The first column describes the feature referred to as "***most common***" in the text, which is the one that completes the question given in the table title, the second column gives the answer, and the third column lists the text reference telling where the answer can be found.

Most Common Feature in Question	*Most Common* Answer	Text Reference
Cause of premenopausal ovarian cystic mass	Functional ovarian cyst (e.g., follicular cysts, corpus luteum cyst)	Chapter 23 I B 1
Type of ovarian epithelial tumors	Serous cystadenomas	Chapter 23 I B 3 a
Type of ovarian germ cell tumors	Benign cystic teratomas (dermoid cysts)	Chapter 23 I B 3 c
Cause of pelvic mass in reproductive years	Pregnancy	Chapter 23 I C 1
Risk factors for ovarian torsion	Ovarian mass size and mobility	Chapter 23 I C 5 a
Symptom of ovarian torsion	Acute, unilateral pelvic pain	Chapter 23 I C 5 b
Risk factor for ovarian cancer	BRCA1 gene	Chapter 23 II A 2
Screening modality for ovarian cancer	Bimanual pelvic examination	Chapter 23 II A 3
Tumor type of ovarian cancer	Epithelial cancer	Chapter 23 II B 1
Primary route of spread of ovarian cancer	Implantation of exfoliated cells via peritoneal fluid circulation	Chapter 23 II B 2
Anatomic site on cervix where dysplasia develops	T-zone	Chapter 24 I A
Risk factor for cervical dysplasia	HPV, types 16 and 18	Chapter 24 I C
Outpatient procedures for destruction of cervical dysplasia	LEEP and cryotherapy	Chapter 24 I I 2, 3
Outcome of untreated mild cervical dysplasia	Spontaneous resolution (65%)	Chapter 24 I E
Tumor type of cervical cancer	Cervical squamous cell carcinoma	Chapter 24 II A 2
Route of spread of cervical cancer	Direct extension	Chapter 24 II C 3
Symptom of cervical cancer	Vaginal bleeding	Chapter 24 II D 1
Symptom of vulvar dystrophy	Vulvar itching	Chapter 25 I B 1
Symptom of vulvar dysplasia	Vulvar itching	Chapter 25 II C 1
Tumor type of vulvar cancer	Vulvar squamous cell carcinoma	Chapter 25 III B 1
Route of spread of vulvar cancer	Direct extension	Chapter 25 III B 3 a
Symptom of vulvar cancer	Vulvar itching	Chapter 25 III C 1
Benign breast condition	Fibrocystic changes	Chapter 26 I A
Benign breast tumor in young women	Fibroadenoma	Chapter 26 I B
Benign cause of blood nipple discharge	Intraductal papilloma	Chapter 26 I E
Nonepithelial neoplasm of the breast	Cystosarcoma phyllodes	Chapter 26 I G
Female malignancy	Breast cancer	Chapter 26 II
Breast malignancy	Infiltrating ductal carcinoma	Chapter 26 II B 1
Sign of Paget's disease of the breast	Pruritic, red, scaly rash involving the nipple	Chapter 26 II B 4
Surgical treatment of choice in early-stage breast cancer	Lumpectomy	Chapter 26 II D 1

Appendix B

Abbreviations

AAS	atypical antibody screen
ACE	angiotensin-converting enzyme
ACTH	adrenocorticotropic hormone
AF	amniotic fluid
AFI	amniotic fluid index
AFP	α-fetoprotein
AIDS	acquired immunodeficiency syndrome
ALT	alanine aminotransferase
AROM	artificial rupture of membranes
ASB	asymptomatic bacteriuria
ASD	atrial septal defect
AST	aspartate aminotransferase
BP	blood pressure
BPD	biparietal diameter
BPP	biophysical profile
BSE	breast self-exam
BSO	bilateral salpingo-oophorectomy
BTB	breakthrough bleeding
BUN	blood urea nitrogen
BV	bacterial vaginosis
CA	carcinoma
CA-125	cancer antigen 125
CAH	congenital adrenal hyperplasia
CBE	clinical breast exam
CEA	carcinoembryonic antigen
CEE	conjugated equine estrogen
CIN	cervical intraepithelial neoplasia
CIS	carcinoma in situ
CMV	cytomegalovirus
CNB	core-needle biopsy
CNS	central nervous system
CPD	cephalopelvic disproportion
CRL	crown–rump length
CS	cesarean section
CST	contraction stress test
CT	computed tomography
CVA	costovertebral angle
CVS	chorionic villus sampling
D&C	dilation and curettage
D&E	dilation and evacuation
DCIS	ductal carcinoma in situ
DES	diethylstilbestrol

DXA	dual-energy x-ray absorptiometry
DHEAS	dehydroepiandrosterone sulfate
DIC	disseminated intravascular coagulation
DM	diabetes mellitus
DST	dexamethasone suppression test
DVT	deep venous thrombosis
ECC	endocervical curettage
EFM	electronic fetal monitoring
EFW	estimated fetal weight
ELISA	enzyme-linked immunosorbent assay
EPCT	estrogen–progesterone challenge test
ERT	estrogen replacement therapy
ESR	erythrocyte sedimentation rate
FBS	fasting blood sugar
FHR	fetal heart rate
FHT	fetal heart tone
FNA	fine-needle aspiration
FSH	follicle-stimulating hormone
FTA-ABS	fluorescent treponema antibody absorption
GBBS	group B β-hemolytic streptococcus
GDM	gestational diabetes mellitus
GI	gastrointestinal
GnRH	gonadotropin-releasing hormone
GTD	gestational trophoblastic disease
HBeAg	hepatitis B e antigen
HBsAg	hepatitis B surface antigen
HBV	hepatitis B virus
hCG	human chorionic gonadotropin
Hct	hematocrit
HDL	high-density lipoprotein
HDN	hemolytic disease of the newborn
HELPP	hemolysis, elevated liver (enzymes), low platelet (count)
Hgb	hemoglobin
HIV	human immunodeficiency virus
hPL	human placental lactogen
HPO	hypothalamic-pituitary-ovarian
HPV	human papilloma virus
HSG	hysterosalpingogram
HSV	herpes simplex virus
HTN	hypertension
ICSI	intracytoplasmic sperm injection
ICU	intensive care unit
IM	intramuscular
IUD	intrauterine device
IUGR	intrauterine growth restriction
IUI	intrauterine insemination
IUT	intrauterine transfusion
IV	intravenous
IVF	in vitro fertilization
IVH	intraventricular hemorrhage
IVP	intravenous pyelogram
LCIS	lobular carcinoma in situ
LDH	lactate dehydrogenase
LDL	low-density lipoprotein
LGV	lymphogranuloma venereum
LEEP	loop electrodiathermy excision procedure
LMP	last menstrual period
L/S	lecithin/sphingomyelin

MCV	mean corpuscular volume
MHA-TP	microhemagglutination assay for *Treponema pallidum*
MIF	müllerian inhibitory factor
MPA	medroxyprogesterone acetate
MRI	magnetic resonance imaging
MS-AFP	maternal serum α-fetoprotein
NEC	necrotizing enterocolitis
NSAID	nonsteroidal anti-inflammatory drug
NST	nonstress test
NTD	neural tube defect
OCP	oral contraceptive pill
OGTT	oral glucose tolerance test
17-OHP	17-OH progesterone
PCOS	polycystic ovarian syndrome
PCR	polymerase chain reaction
PCT	progesterone challenge test
PDA	patent ductus arteriosus
PID	pelvic inflammatory disease
PIH	pregnancy-induced hypertension
PMS	premenstrual syndrome
PO	oral
POC	products of conception
PPD	postpartum day
PPH	postpartum hemorrhage
PROM	premature rupture of membranes
PT	prothrombin time
PTT	partial thromboplastin time
PTU	propylthiouracil
PUBS	percutaneous umbilical blood sampling
PUPPP	pruritic urticarial papules and pustules of pregnancy
RBC	red blood cell
RDS	respiratory distress syndrome
ROP	retinopathy of prematurity
RPR	rapid plasma reagin (test)
RT	radiation therapy
SBE	subacute bacterial endocarditis
SERM	selective estrogen receptor modulator
SIL	squamous intraepithelial lesion
SLE	systemic lupus erythematosus
SPROM	spontaneous premature rupture of membranes
SSRI	selective serotonin reuptake inhibitor
STD	sexually transmitted disease
TAH	total abdominal hysterectomy
TOA	tubo-ovarian abscess
TSH	thyroid-stimulating hormone
T (zone)	transformation (zone)
UA	urinalysis
UC	uterine contraction
URI	upper respiratory infection
UTI	urinary tract infection
VAS	vibroacoustic stimulation
VBAC	vaginal birth after cesarean
VDRL	Venereal Disease Research Laboratory (test)
VIN	vulvar intraepithelial neoplasia
VSD	ventricular septal defect
WBC	white blood cell

Index

Page numbers in *italics* denote figures; those followed by "t" denote tables